Oral Communication Problems in Children and Adolescents

Edited by

Sol Adler, Ph.D.

Professor and Director
Pediatric Language Programs
Department of Audiology and Speech Pathology
The University of Tennessee
Knoxville, Tennessee

 Grune & Stratton   1988

An Imprint of the W. B. Saunders Company
Harcourt Brace Jovanovich, Publishers

Philadelphia San Diego London Toronto
Montreal Sydney Tokyo

Oral communication problems in children and
adolescents.

Includes index.
1. Learning disabled children—Education—United
States.   2. Learning disabled youth—education—
United States.   3. Oral communication—United States.
4. Language disorders in children—United States.
I. Adler, Sol, 1925–
LC4704.5.073   1987   371.9'0973   87–25024
ISBN 0–8089–1887–7

Grune & Stratton
Philadelphia, PA 19105

Library of Congress Catalog Number 87-25024
International Standard Book Number 0–8089–1887–7
Printed in the United States of America

87 88 89 90   10 9 8 7 6 5 4 3 2 1

Contents

Preface

For many years we have taught teachers and prospective teachers about the numerous problems that occur to children who possess oral communication disorders; in addition, we have presented information concerning the role the teacher should play in the treatment of these disorders and concomitant problems. Our interactions and experiences with teachers and student teachers have demonstrated the need for a textbook that incorporates such information: a book that is comprehensive yet devoid of professional jargon, intermediate between the complex text available for classroom adoption and the simplistic and brief treatise. We believe that teachers with knowledge of different speech–language–hearing deficiencies can have a major impact on the successful remediation of these disorders.

Authors with expertise in the specific subject matter they address have been asked to write the various chapters. We have asked them to keep in mind the needs of the student teachers and the classroom teachers as they write their chapters. If, by serendipity, others, and particularly parents, can profit from reading these materials, then we are pleased.

Our fundamental aim in preparing this book is to inform teachers and prospective teachers, as well as to aid them in their classroom responsibilities to children or adolescents who may happen to stutter, possess voice, articulation, or language deficiencies, manifest hearing problems, or use cultural speech–language patterns. We believe it to be patently true that such information will (1) enable teachers to be of significant help in the speech–language pathologist's (SLP)* remediation program, and (2) help teachers to avoid harmful blunders in their interactions with these children. Such mistakes may have a dramatic effect upon the child.

For example, my first recollection of being a stutterer occurred when I was told by my third grade teacher, "Do not talk like that." Heretofore, I had not been aware of any speech disturbance. After her persistent comments, however, I recognized that my speech was, in fact, different from the speech of other children in the classroom.

Teachers must be taught the "dos and don'ts" insofar as stuttering and other disorders are concerned. Teachers must recognize that in conjunction with the SLP and the parent(s), they may play a very beneficial role in helping communicatively

---

* We use the terms speech–language clinician and speech–language pathologist synonymously throughout the book.

impaired pupils—or, conversely, they may create more problems for them. However, we must remember that the teacher's prime responsibility is to teach and not to remediate. We hope to give them intelligible information that is useful but not burdensome in the classroom.

We have solicited information that will be helpful to teachers. We hope we have succeeded in this endeavor.

Introduction

THE POPULATION TO WHOM THIS BOOK IS DIRECTED: THE TEACHERS

We envision that this book will be used as a text (1) in those academic classes designed to acquaint education majors or special education majors with the dynamics of aural-oral communication disorders, or (2) by practicing teachers who desire an enhanced understanding of the speech–language–hearing disordered children or adolescents in their classrooms. We believe this textbook will also serve the needs of professionals in recertification workshops, pre-service or in-service programs, and/or other short-term continuing education programs. We stress the teachers' role regarding the pupils in their classes who happen to possess some kind of communicative disorder. We also have tried to use language that is meaningful to the teacher, eliminating much professional jargon.

What are the "dos and don'ts"? What is the teacher's role? What should teachers do for children in their classes who stutter, who "don't talk plain," who possess any of the other disorders discussed in the book? What can the teacher do to prevent the occurrence of such disorders? What is the teacher's role *vis-a-vis* the SLP—or the parent(s) of speech–language–hearing disordered children? These questions and others are discussed.

As noted in the preface, we have taught teachers in recertification workshops for many years. There is little question that these professional workshops can provide enormous help in the therapeutic enhancement of children's speech and language skills. Conversely, it is equally apparent that with insufficient understanding of aural-oral communication processes, the teachers can prove to be a significant detriment to the therapy program.

It is important that the teachers and the SLPs have mutual understanding and respect for their respective disciplines. According to the American Speech-Language-Hearing Association (1964), the consultant function of the SLP has played a vital role in the provision of equal education for all handicapped individuals. The SLP in the public schools should help to devise and implement programs for classroom use and educate the classroom teachers and administrators in the identification, management, and prevention of communication disorders. The chapters in this book have been assembled for these purposes.

In Part I, detailed introductory information for the reader is presented. For those who want only a relatively simplistic overview of aural-oral disorders, it is recommended that they read this first part of the book.

In Part II, the various contributors to the book present detailed information. Drs. Robinson and Brown discuss the kinds of language deficiencies often heard in children as well as the causes and suggested treatment for these problems. The following chapter pertains to language differences in children—nonstandard dialectal speech patterns—and is written by Dr. Bountress, a recognized authority. Drs. Mary H. Pannbacker and Grace P. Middleton discuss the different voice problems frequently heard in children. The insidious effects of stuttering are addressed by Dr. Theodore Mandel!. Rhonda Work, a former member of the American Speech-Language-Hearing Association executive board and well known for her expertise, discusses the most common of all disorders—articulation. Finally, Drs. Diefendorf and Leverett, in the last two chapters, present information regarding hearing impairment and aural disorders in children: causation, assessment, and treatment, followed by data concerning the educational management of the hearing-impaired child.

Contributors

Nicholas G. Bountress, Ed.D.
Professor
Speech Pathology and Audiology
Child Study Center
Old Dominion University
Norfolk, Virginia

Asa J. Brown, Ph.D.
Professor and Head
Department of Special Education
Wayne State University
Detroit, Michigan

Allan O. Diefendorf, Ph.D.
Associate Professor
Department of Audiology and Speech Pathology
University of Tennessee
Knoxville, Tennessee

Ralph G. Leverett, Ph.D.
Professor
Department of Education and Psychology
Trevecca Nazarene College
Nashville, Tennessee

Theodore Mandell, Ed.D.
Supervisor (Retired)
Department of Communication Disorders
Detroit Public Schools; and
Adjunct Professor of Special Education
Wayne State University
Detroit, Michigan

Grace F. Middleton, Ed.D.
Assistant Professor
Program in Speech, Hearing and Language Disorders
College of Nursing and Allied Health
University of Texas
El Paso, Texas

Mary H. Pannbacker, Ph.D.
Professor and Program Director
Department of Communication Disorders
School of Allied Health Professions
Louisiana State University Medical Center
Shreveport, Louisiana

Jane E. Robinson, Ph. D.
Assistant Professor and School Practicum Coordinator
Department of Audiology and Speech Pathology
Department of Special Education and Rehabilitation
University of Tennessee
Knoxville, Tennessee

Rhonda S. Work, M.A.
Program Specialist Supervisor
Bureau of Education for Exceptional Students
Florida Department of Education
Tallahassee, Florida

PART I

General Information for the Teacher

1

An Introduction to Communicative Behavior

Sol Adler

We live in a talking world. Feelings, thoughts, ideas, and information constantly are conveyed by audible symbols. The child's or adolescent's various aural-oral communicative needs are expressed as follows.

SPEECH-LANGUAGE-HEARING DISORDERS/DIFFERENCES

Speech Disorders

Speech refers to the transmission of language symbols—the voice and rhythm components of oral communication. There are a variety of voice disorders, all of which are very prevalent in school-age children. The rhythm disorder, otherwise known as stuttering, is not as common as the diverse voice problems, but is more insidious in its effects.

Articulation Disorders

The most common of the oral communication disorders, articulatory deficiency comprises approximately 85–90 percent of the caseloads for many public school speech–language clinicians. There is much the classroom teacher can do to help these children, particularly those in K-2 grades.

Language Disorders

Language problems are subdivided into categories according to their major causes: minimal brain dysfunction, mental retardation, autism, emotional disturbances, and environmental causes. By *language* we refer to the phonemes or sounds, the vocabulary or lexicon, the grammar or the syntax and morphology, and the

ORAL COMMUNICATION PROBLEMS
IN CHILDREN AND ADOLESCENTS
Copyright © 1988 by Grune & Stratton, Inc.

ISBN 0-8089-1887-7
All rights reserved.

pragmatics or the way language is used by children in different situations and contexts, for example, children initiating or terminating conversation in the classroom and/or in the home. The first named language unit, phonemes or sounds (articulation), is covered in a separate chapter due to its prevalence as a disorder in school-age children.

Many children with language disorders possess some kind of developmental disability. *Developmental disability* is a term reflecting impaired abilities in young children. Common types of developmental disability are cerebral palsy, mental retardation, blindness, deafness, autism, etc. (see Chapter 2). In past years, these children frequently were placed in segregated environments. Today, due to PL 94-142 (1975),* and its mandate that children be mainstreamed if at all possible (i.e., least-restrictive environment), a number of exceptional children are situated for the full day, or part of the day, in the regular classroom or resource room. Classroom teachers need to have some relevant information about the problems possessed by these children if they are to relate effectively to them.

Language Differences

Social dialects, such as black English and appalachian English,† are rule-governed and nonstandard dialectal patterns used by many lower-class poor students. The impact that these dialectal patterns have upon education and employment opportunities is profound.

Hearing Disorders

There are different types and severity levels of hearing losses. If undetected, hearing problems can cause significant language and learning disorders to occur. The educational audiologist—a specialist trained to test for hearing loss, to train residual auditory function, and to maximize hearing through amplification (the hearing aid)— may be a member of the public school staff.

To understand what is heard, the child must process the auditory or aural input; thus children must not only hear what is said, they must also pay attention, retain, perceive, and sequence that which they hear. These functions are commonly labeled *auditory* or *aural processing skills*. A deficiency in any one or more of these skills will result in impaired receptive language as well as inability to follow or carry out directions appropriate to classroom behavior.

---

* This law mandates that *all* exceptional children regardless of the severity or nature of their exceptionality must receive an appropriate education. Many of these children also possess a concomitant communicative disorder. A more current law (PL99-457, 1987) extends these services to infants and toddlers.

† Although many writers capitalize the words "black" and "appalachian," we see no valid reason to do so.

NORMAL VERSUS ABNORMAL COMMUNICATIVE BEHAVIOR IN CHILDREN

Although many experienced teachers can readily distinguish between most normal and abnormal utterances, it would be useful to present some information pertinent to that which is normal before we discuss the abnormalities of speech–language–hearing behavior.

Speech

Voice patterns should be firmly established by the time the child is in the early elementary grades. The pitch used should be appropriate for the age. Both boys and girls possess very similar pitches in K-1; it is only as they grow older that stature alters the males' pitch usage. Thus the pitch used should be neither too high nor too low relevant to the age, sex, and body size of the child or adolescent. Similarly, the loudness level should be appropriate for the typical verbal activities that take place in the classroom, being neither too loud nor too soft. Finally, voice quality should be pleasing to the ear; it should not be marred by chronic hoarseness or harshness, or too much or too little nasality.

Abnormal speech rhythms or stuttering may develop differently in children. For example, at about the age of 2 1/2–3 years of age, children's speech rhythm is disturbed by repetitions and other minimal disturbances in speech patterns. This same disturbance is again noticed when children enter school or are in the K-1 grades. Many of these children with repetitions will outgrow the hesitancies and interruptions in their speech rhythm, while other children will become stutterers.

Articulation

The child's ability to say correctly the different sounds of our language occurs as a function of maturational development as well as the amount and type of speech stimulation received by the child. More specifically, because of the genetic differences inherent in children—some of them mature earlier or later than others—or because of the nature of the speech stimulation they receive in the home or from peer associations, some children say their sounds correctly earlier or later in life than others. Thus, the later appearing sounds such as /s/, /z/, /th/, /l/, and /r/ may appear consistently correct in the speech of some children in K-1 but not in the speech used by all of the children. For those latter children, stimulation activities would be most useful in helping them to develop these skills. For children who still manifest articulation errors in the second grade, there should be careful examinations made as to the reason for the errors. It may be of some pathologic significance that requires the attention of the speech–language pathologist.

Language

Children in the early elementary grades are usually loquacious—they talk a lot. Since most children have approximately 90 percent of their grammatical skills intact by the time they are 5 years of age, they should be using fairly good syntactic and morphological utterances. Their vocabulary should also be sufficiently large to allow for diversified expressions. If either their grammar or vocabulary appears to be impoverished, it may be due to a pathology (e.g., minimal brain dysfunction) and should receive the attention of the speech–language pathologist. They must also be able to properly initiate and terminate conversations; that is, to use language that is appropriate to the situation (i.e., the pragmatics of language).

Hearing

Auditory acuity, attention, retention, discrimination, and sequencing skills are of fundamental importance to the development of appropriate communication skills and desirable learning habits. For example, acceptable selective attention and normal retentive abilities are of obvious importance. Yet, relatively little importance is placed upon the development of these skills as compared to the time and effort teachers normally spend on visual perceptual training.

In the typical kindergarten class about half the children will be easily distracted, that is, possess poor selective attention, and manifest a "leaky bucket" syndrome (the possession of poor retentive abilities). In the first and second grades, the number of children with these deficiencies gradually will be attenuated so that only a few children may still manifest these problems. Our rule of thumb is that any third grader who still presents such auditory processing disturbances probably possesses a pathology of the processing system and should receive an evaluation by the speech–language pathologist.

SOME COMMON COMMUNICATION DISORDERS

A traditional definition of a speech disorder involves a judgment on the part of the listener as to whether or not the child's speech differs significantly and sufficiently from the norm to call attention to itself—to be conspicuous. What then is the norm? Simplistically, it is what is to be expected considering the child's age and cultural background. Thus, there is no universal norm because of different sociolinguistic-cultural heritages.

In evaluating the speech of pupils in the classroom, the following checklist will be found to be useful. If the teacher notices that a child possesses one or more of these disorders and is not receiving speech therapy, an immediate referral should be made to the speech–language pathologist.

Speech Disorders
Voice Disorders
1. Pitch is too high or too low for the child's sex, age, stature.
2. Loudness (too loud or too soft) is not relevant to the speaking environment.
3. Voice quality is either hyper- or hyponasal; there is chronic hoarseness or harshness.

Stuttering
1. There are abnormal repetitions and/or prolongations of sounds, syllables, and/or words.
2. There are facial and/or bodily grimaces and/or contortions while stuttering.
3. There is obvious embarrassment while stuttering.

Articulation
1. Sounds are omitted, added, distorted, or substituted.
2. The child is difficult to understand.

Language Disorders
The pupil manifests
1. limited vocabulary;
2. disordered syntax;
3. writing and/or reading disorders;
4. impoverished thought or judgmental abilities or ability to express oneself properly (i.e., to "stay on topic," or change topic as is appropriate);
5. poor turn-taking skills regarding the initiation or termination of a conversation.

Language Differences
1. The student uses what is commonly termed a social dialect: mountain English, black English, hispanic English.

Hearing Disorders
1. There are changes in customary hearing behavior, general behavior, or learning skills. There may be poor selective attention or retention of directions.

2

A Brief Overview of some of the Different Exceptionalities—Disorders Encountered in the Classroom

Sol Adler

Children possessing any one or more of the following disorders may manifest a deficiency in their aural-oral communication skills.

CLEFT LIP AND/OR PALATE

The cleft of the lip (sometimes called "hare-lip") and/or palate will occur during the third month of pregnancy. The causes of the cleft condition may be genetic or teratogenic: this latter term pertains to some deleterious influence that occurs after normal conception; for example, certain illnesses, drugs, or X rays during the first trimester may cause an abnormality to occur in the fetus' development.

Clefts of the lip may be unilateral or bilateral. In any case, the cleft(s) usually is surgically repaired before the infant leaves the hospital and therefore the cleft(s) has no impact upon the emergent oral behavior of the child.

Clefts of the palate are of diverse types and are more serious: they will negatively affect the oral behavior of the child. These clefts usually are closed sometime between 2–3 years of age. As a result of this disorder, the child may manifest both articulation and nasality deficiencies. Many of these children also have frequent bouts with conductive type hearing loss, and therefore their auditory acuity must be carefully monitored.

ORAL COMMUNICATION PROBLEMS
IN CHILDREN AND ADOLESCENTS
Copyright © 1988 by Grune & Stratton, Inc.

ISBN 0-8089-1887-7
All rights reserved.

CEREBRAL PALSY

Cerebral palsy is a neuromuscular disorder (preferred term) that is caused by an insult (damage) to the brain before, during, or after birth that negatively affects the child's muscular movements. Intelligence may or may not be impaired; many such children possess high IQs. Whether or not articulation and voice quality disorders are present is dependent on the muscles affected. For example, if the muscles responsible for articulation are impaired, there will be an articulatory disorder, and this disorder is known by a special name—dysarthria.

There are three major types of cerebral palsy: (1) Tonus disorders are characterized by spasticity or flaccidity. By tonus disorder we refer to an impairment in the electrical transmission system of the nerves leading from the damaged brain; by spasticity, we refer to a muscle that is "tight" or spastic; and conversely, by flaccidity we mean a muscle state that is the opposite of spasticity—a limpness of the muscle. Tonus disorders can affect the legs only (paraplegia), the legs mainly and the arms slightly (diplegia), one side of the body (hemiplegia), all four limbs (quadriplegia). These paralyses or pareses (mild paralyses) are of different severity levels and may or may not affect the muscles involved in speech production. These muscular systems are: (*a*) respiration or the air supply necessary for sound production, (*b*) phonation or voicing of the sound, (*c*) resonation or amplification of selected sound frequencies, and (*d*) articulation or the production of the sounds. (2) Athetosis is characterized by a constant squirming or writhing motion. The arms and upper torso, in particular, are in constant motion. (3) Ataxia is characterized by incoordination between the flexor and extensor muscles. Specifically, each movement one makes is a product of both flexor and extensor (sometimes named agonist and antagonist) muscle components; for example, when a person opens the mouth, the flexor muscles contract and the extensors relax; as the mouth is closed, the flexors now relax and the extensors contract. The contractions and relaxations of the paired muscle groups have to occur coordinately if the movement is to be appropriate. In ataxia, the damage to the cerebellum of the brain does not allow for the proper coordination of the paired muscles. If the uncoordinated movements occur in the muscles of respiration, phonation, resonation, and/or articulation, a speech disorder will result.

TONSILLECTOMY AND ADENOIDECTOMY (T & A)

The tonsils and adenoids usually achieve their maximum growth during the time the child is in the first and second grades; following this time span the tonsils and adenoids frequently decrease in size and no longer are problems.

Enlarged tonsils and adenoids can cause a variety of problems: (1) the tonsils may cause swallowing to be a relatively painful act; (2) the adenoids may (*a*) block the Eustachian tube located in the back of the throat and impair its ability to transmit an appropriate air supply and air pressure to the middle ear, thus causing pain and possible pathology to the ear; or (*b*) block the air supply from entering the nasal channels in the back of the pharynx or throat and causing hyponasality. In past years, the enlarged tonsils and adenoids were rather routinely removed; today, because of our knowledge concerning their ability to manufacture white blood cells, the tonsils and adenoids are removed only if necessary.

When a T & A is performed, it is the absence of the adenoids that may create a problem—hopefully, only a temporary hypernasal voice quality. After about a month or so following their excision, the voice quality usually reverts back to normal. The removal of the tonsils generally does not cause any kind of speech problem.

TONGUE-TIE

At the birth of the infant, the physician will routinely examine the status of the lingual (tongue) frenum (tie) to determine if it is abnormal and interferes with tongue-tip mobility. If so, it is clipped and appropriate movement is attained. Thus, all people are born with a tongue-tie but only a few possess an abnormal lingual frenum.

Occasionally an atypical tongue-tie condition persists into childhood and will be manifested by (1) poor tongue-tip movement, as when licking a sucker or ice cream cone, and (2) substandard articulation of those sounds involving the tongue-tip, such as /t/ and /d/ when rapid transitions of the tongue are required as in connected speech patterns.

THE MENTALLY RETARDED (MR) VERSUS THE FUNCTIONALLY RETARDED (FR) CHILD

The MR child is unable to perform appropriately (normally) on both standardized intelligence tests and adaptive behavior tests (i.e., a measure of the individual's knowledge of essential skills), for example, appropriate use of the telephone, using money properly, etc. Either genetic causes or brain damage sustained before, during, or after birth may result in this condition.

The FR child performs inappropriately on IQ tests but normally on tests of adaptive behavior. These children are almost always culturally different and poor. Because they are not MR, they do not belong in programs designed for the MR (e.g., in past years, the classroom for the educable mentally retarded [EMR] was comprised mainly of FR children. These children perform poorly on IQ tests because of the cultural bias inherent in the test (poor test validity), and/or because of inappropriate testing procedures (poor test reliability).

MR children will possess a language retardation—an impoverishment of linguistic information; FR children will possess a language difference—a sufficiency of linguistic information but in their own dialect.

3

General Guidelines for the Teacher

Sol Adler

BE A GOOD SPEECH MODEL

The touchstone of educational acquisition is effective communication: conversely, an impaired ability to understand or to transmit aural-oral information will often interfere with the development of the basic academic skills such as reading, writing, and spelling. There is much the teacher can do to enhance communicative skills development in young children.

Five simple but important examples are as follows:

1. Create a verbally permissive environment in the classroom by rewarding all attempts at communication by children who tend to be nonparticipants. The communicatively disordered child frequently falls into this category.
2. Be a good listener. When a child talks make it quite obvious that you are paying attention to the comments.
3. Simplify your utterances: make them shorter and simpler.
4. Enhance your speech prosody (inflections, stress, and in general, speech rhythm) when talking to children.
5. Use much bodily movement to accompany your speech; the more you use your hands and body in rhythm with your speech utterances, the more effective will be your classroom interactions with the children.

All teachers, particularly in K-2, need to be aware of the importance of appropriate standard English usage when talking to the children in their classrooms. Their oral communication pattern frequently serves as a model for these children, especially younger ones. A teacher with a lisp, for example, may cause children in the K-2 grades to imitate the speech defect and thus making it a chronic problem.

ORAL COMMUNICATION PROBLEMS
IN CHILDREN AND ADOLESCENTS
Copyright © 1988 by Grune & Stratton, Inc.

ISBN 0-8089-1887-7
All rights reserved.

INDIRECT LANGUAGE STIMULATION TECHNIQUES FOR PRESCHOOL-AGE CHILDREN IN THE HOME, DAY CARE, OR NURSERY PROGRAM

As more and more children are enrolled in preschool education programs, it becomes increasingly clear that the teachers or aides in these programs should be capable of providing appropriate types or amounts of linguistic stimulation to the children.

Receptive Language.   How we understand what we hear; the decoding of words.

For example: "The sky is *blue.*
"Daddy is wearing a *blue* tie."

Preschool aged children must learn the word "blue" in its various usages. Older children must learn to decode more abstract words.

Expressive Language.   How we use linguistic symbols or words with concomitant speech prosody (inflections, stress patterns, etc.). We can help children learn to use language more efficiently by the following:

1. *Child centered parallel talk.* The adult describes what the child is doing as the youngster does it, for example, "You're rolling the ball."
2. *Object centered descriptive talk.* The adult provides word labels for the objects the child is playing with, for example, "The ball is rolling."
3. *Self-talk.* The adult talks about an action as the child watches, for example, "I'm washing the dish; now I'm drying the dish."

There should be concern among teachers regarding the development of desirable speech–language behavior in their pupils. By being a good speech model, the teacher can significantly enhance students' oral behavior.

DISTINGUISH AMONG STANDARD, NONSTANDARD, AND SUBSTANDARD SPEECH PATTERNS

It is important that a bidialectal communications (see Chapter 9) program be developed for those children who speak in social dialects, such as mountain or black English. All teachers should be aware of the distinction between standard, nonstandard, and substandard communication. That which is incorrect or substandard should be eradicated by overt or covert correction; that is, if a middle class child says something that is patently substandard, the teacher can say to the child "What you said is incorrect. It should be said as follows . . . " Or the teacher may repeat what the child uttered but say it in correct standard English. This constant attention to children's speech–language patterns ultimately will convince them of the desirability of speaking in correct standard English.

ENHANCE AUDITORY PROCESSING TRAINING IN K-1

Develop an extensive auditory processing program for the young child. In this era of television watching, children's auditory skills have been neglected. It has been our experience that kindergarten teachers spend more time with visual processing tasks in preparation for reading and writing development than with the more basic and fundamental auditory tasks such as: attention, retention, sequencing, recognition and discrimination, and concept development.

ENHANCE ORAL COMMUNICATION IN K-12

Teach children to become effective oral communicators. This can be accomplished only if there is concern among teachers for the development of oral communication abilities in children. This concern can be readily and easily translated into an effective program by giving each pupil an opportunity to present short speeches (e.g., "Show and Tell" in early grades) to classmates, and then be critiqued by the teacher regarding the content and the dynamics of the presentation; that is, how effective was the child's transmission of the information.

DIALOGUE WITH THE COMMUNICATIVELY DISORDERED CHILD

Initiate a dialogue with those children possessing disordered oral communication skills. Discuss the apparent problem with the child or adolescent. What are the pupil's needs, problems? Can the teacher help the child? If in fact the pupil has a disorder, there should be a concerted effort on the part of the clinician, the parent, and the teacher to set in motion a remedial program to which all can contribute in their own time and way.

Clearly there are some activities that should be the province of only the clinician, but there are many ways the teacher and parent can work in conjunction with the clinician to enhance the child's therapeutic progress.

THE INTERRELATIONSHIP BETWEEN THE SPEECH PERFORMANCE AND THE PERSONALITY

Recognize that speech–language–hearing disorders can have a very deleterious effect upon a child's psyche and self-concept, that is, the personality development of the child. Untreated communication disorders or improperly or unsuccessfully treated problems can cause its possessor to develop a poor self-concept, a weak psyche, and, in general, an unhealthy personality. A significant interrelationship exists between our speech patterns and our feelings about ourselves; teachers should recognize, therefore, the necessity to react positively to these problems and not to ignore them.

4

The Speech-Language Pathologist

Sol Adler

Informal surveys of teachers and of teacher preparation curricula, of which an aural-oral communicative disorders course is a part, show that although many institutions of higher learning offer such a course, many teachers graduate with little understanding of these disorders. They may have received some didactic information concerning the various speech–language problems manifested by school-age populations, but relatively little understanding of their relationship to these children or adolescents.

Teachers of both normal and exceptional children (i.e., special educators) need to understand what their roles are vis-à-vis the speech–language defective child, the nature of the impact teachers may have upon such children, what teachers can do to help in the remedial program, and how and why they should collaborate with both the speech–language pathologist and the parent in an attempt to fashion an optimum habilitative program for each child. Basic to this interrelationship is an understanding of the role of the speech–language pathologist.

THE PUBLIC SCHOOL SPEECH-LANGUAGE PATHOLOGIST AND THE THERAPY PROGRAM

It is incumbent on teachers to recognize that the qualifications of different speech–language pathologists may differ significantly as a function of their educational training and clinical experience. As with most other professional workers, the speech–language pathologist may possess a bachelor's degree with limited previous clinical practicum—mainly with children possessing articulation disorders. Or, the speech–language pathologist may have earned a master's or doctorate degree with significant hours of clinical practicum with a host of children and adults possessing differing communicative disorders.

ORAL COMMUNICATION PROBLEMS
IN CHILDREN AND ADOLESCENTS
Copyright © 1988 by Grune & Stratton, Inc.

ISBN 0-8089-1887-7
All rights reserved.

The teacher should recognize that the American Speech–Language Hearing Association (ASHA) certifies its members—gives its Certificate of Clinical Competence (CCC)in either speech–language pathology or audiology. Some members possess the CCC in both areas of expertise. A speech–language pathologist who possesses such certification has not only a master's degree from an accredited college or university training program, and a significant number of practicum hours, but also has served a 9-month internship (fellowship year) and successfully completed a qualifying examination.

Some speech–language pathologists who are members of ASHA, may be more generalists than specialists. Since more difficult cases may require the attention of a highly trained specialist, the school teacher should not expect every communicatively disordered child to be effectively treated by the speech–language pathologist; there are times when referrals to other practitioners in private practice or college or university training centers may be required.

Clearly any child who has received therapy for a number of years without significant progress should be examined by such a specialist. Perhaps a new and a fresh approach will be indicated. This decision making should be a joint process involving all adult interactors in the child's program. It should be noted, however, that when such referrals are made, the school system, and not the parents, is often liable for the cost of the examination.

THE THERAPY PROTOCOL

Because of financial limitation, some school systems employ few speech–language pathologists thus forcing clinicians to handle large caseloads. By doing this they can see each child only once or twice a week for very limited amounts of time. Such a protocol is obviously self-limiting if the child in question possesses a significant disorder requiring more time and more frequent interaction than possible under the conventional format. Frequently, it is for this reason that some children are treated unsuccessfully in long-term school therapy programs.

There are, however, school systems that have been able to develop protocols that allow for intensive therapeutic interactions for children with significant problems. The speech–language pathologists who interact with these children have a much smaller caseload and can therefore treat them more frequently and for increased time units.

THE TITLE: WHAT TO CALL THE SPEECH–LANGUAGE PATHOLOGIST

Our preferred term is speech–language pathologist or clinician. However, the speech–language pathologist goes by a variety of names of which perhaps the most common are speech teacher or speech therapist.

THE NATURE OF THE RELATIONSHIP—TEACHER-SPEECH- LANGUAGE PATHOLOGIST-PARENT

There must be an effective interrelationship, particularly between the teacher and the speech–language pathologist, if children are to make the kind of progress they frequently are capable of making. The reason for this lack of appropriate progress may stem from a paucity of appropriate and sufficient "carryover" programs in the classroom and in the home. Most children can benefit from the treatment offered by the speech–language pathologist inside the therapy room. They have problems, however, in remembering to use their new speech–language skills outside the therapy room. By having the teacher and parent cooperate in this carryover process from therapy room to classroom to home, much additional progress can be made.

Both teachers and speech–language pathologists often are inundated with academic meetings, interactions with parents, and especially paperwork, plus a variety of other duties frequently assigned to them. This inundation prevents the kind of cooperative relationship between these professional workers that is so relevant and important to the children who possess communicative disorders. We believe that all teachers, who have children in their classrooms receiving therapy, should be informed as to the nature of the child's problem and the therapy progress of each child. In particular, there should be time for a discussion as to what they, the teachers, can to to expedite the therapy progress of the children.

How and when such conferences are to be held is not germane; time must be found for such interactions if the child in question is not only to be helped but also not to be hurt due to teacher misinformation regarding a particular disorder. For example, one teacher—a devoted and kind person—was convinced that the stuttering boy in her fifth grade class could and would be helped if, as Demosthenes did, he kept pebbles in his mouth as he talked in class. The shame experienced by this boy was significantly enhanced by this teacher.

We would urge speech–language pathologists to present in-service workshops to teachers, and teachers to request such workshops. Through this medium much misinformation can be corrected, and much new information can be provided.

When possible, parental cooperation should be sought so that all adults who interact with communicatively impaired children relate to them in a similar manner, with similar goals, and with similar methods for reaching the goals.

COOPERATIVE SPECIFICS

Cooperation between the teacher and clinician should be maximal, rather than minimal. For example, it would be helpful if the teacher:

1. had some understanding of the methods and techniques being employed by the clinician. This obviously requires that the clinician and teacher find time to interact—to talk—about these matters;

2. could furnish the clinician with periodic reports on the child's progress in the classroom and vice versa in the therapy room;‡
3. maintain good motivation, morale, and self-concept in the child. In part, this is accomplished by not allowing other children to imitate, make fun of, or ridicule the speech defective child.

THE SPEECH-LANGUAGE PATHOLOGIST

If you are a teacher of K-1, suggest that the speech–language pathologist spend approximately 20 minutes, twice a week, developing a speech improvement program in your class. If possible, have the clinician use your readers and/or materials to demonstrate the effectiveness of this kind of improvement program. So many of the children on the caseload of the clinician come from K-1 classes that it is patently proper for the speech–language pathologist to find the time to do this kind of activity. It is mutually helpful. On the one hand, such speech improvement programs can eliminate by 30–40 percent or more the size of the clinician's caseload; on the other hand, it can demonstrate to the teacher the many helpful aural-oral activities that may be utilized in the classroom.

Most speech–language pathologists interact with communicatively impaired children in three or four schools. It is logistically feasible for most of these clinicians to find the time to perform such classroom activities, particularly when it allows for a sizeable reduction in interactions with children needing articulation stimulation and possessing, for the most part, articulation disorders. This reduction in caseload will enable the clinician to work more intensively with the children possessing more severe disorders.

The significance of this relationship to both the clinician and teacher deserves to be underscored. We can only speculate as to why such interactions are not more common, but we can dogmatically state that the benefits to be accrued by the pupils as well as the participants—the teacher and the clinician—are manifold.

THE SPEECH-LANGUAGE PATHOLOGIST IN OTHER CLASSROOMS

The speech–language pathologist should spend some time in classes other than K-1, particularly the self-contained class for handicapped children and the resource room for less severely affected children. So many of these children possess auditory processing and oral expressive language problems, as well as articulation disorders, that it would be time well spent in helping the children and demonstrating the kinds of aural-oral activities useful in such classes.

---

‡ In some school systems, speech–language pathologists have to send out progress reports to the teachers every 6 weeks.

It would also be appropriate for the clinician to visit other elementary, middle school, and high school classes as time permits and as teachers' requests for such activities are made. If a teacher believes such presentations in the classroom would be helpful, a request should be made of the speech–language pathologist. This is particularly the case in schools that contain mostly rural or black children or lower-class children from other ethnic, racial, or cultural groups who speak primarily in a social dialect. Some speech–language pathologists can be of much help in developing bidialectal-bicultural lesson plans for the classroom.

5

The Teacher, Parent, Speech-Language Clinician Interaction

Sol Adler

UNDERSTANDING THE PROBLEMS OF THE CHILD AND HOW THEY MAY IMPACT ON THE FAMILY: LISTENING TO THE PARENTS

Close attention should be given to the negative impact that an exceptional child may have upon the family constellation. Speech and/or hearing handicapped children may cause much trauma to occur within the family unit. To understand these problems—the affective and financial problems—the teacher and speech-language clinician must listen carefully not only to what the parent(s) say, but the nature of any underlying distress they may covertly convey.

LISTENING TO EACH OTHER: WHAT ARE THE PROBLEMS EACH OF THE PROFESSIONAL WORKERS MAY HAVE WITH THE CHILD OR WITH THE PARENTS OF THE CHILD?

The exceptional child and/or the parents may create problems for either or both the teacher and speech–language clinician. To obviate these problems and to eliminate discord between these professional workers, each should know what the other has said or recommended to such children and/or their parents. Working in a vacuum whereby the speech–language clinician does not inform the teacher, or vice versa, does not contribute to a unified approach to the problem(s).

ORAL COMMUNICATION PROBLEMS
IN CHILDREN AND ADOLESCENTS
Copyright © 1988 by Grune & Stratton, Inc.

PUBLIC LAW 94-142: MAINSTREAMING AND THE LEAST RESTRICTIVE ENVIRONMENT

Many children and adolescents with a variety of different developmental disabilities also possess aural-oral communication disorders. It is important that the teacher understand the ramifications of this law as it pertains to mainstreaming or the integration of both normal and handicapped children in a classroom environment that is optimally helpful or conversely least restrictive to the exceptional children. Placement of such children in segregated environments is appropriate only when the M-Team (the Multidisciplinary Team) comprised of at least three members: the principal or a surrogate—the teacher, the parent, and one other member—often the school psychologist and/or the speech–language clinician decides that such placement is necessary for suitable learning to occur. However, when it is possible for the child to participate in the regular classroom environment and/or a resource room, such placement should occur. If this is the proper course of action, support must be given to the classroom teacher by the administration and the professional workers concerned with the child's problem.

Mainstreaming is generally not very effective, or at least as effective as it might be, due to lack of teacher support or guidance. We should not expect teachers with minimal training in the various developmental disabilities, the mentally retarded, the seizure disordered, the neuromuscular impaired (e.g., cerebral palsied), etc. to know how to teach these individuals. Practical suggestions must be given to teachers regarding optimum teaching and behavior management strategies. The introduction of an intermediary between the classroom teacher and the special teacher and/ or the speech–language clinician would also be most helpful.

THE SCHOOL M-TEAM

Services for communicatively handicapped children in public schools have increased in both the numbers being served and in the sophistication of the diagnostic and treatment programs. Concomitant with the increase of these services has been an enhanced awareness of the need for school personnel, particularly teachers, to participate in program planning for these children—a M-Team approach to planning.

Since aural-oral disorders are often one symptom of a syndrome manifested by an exceptional child with a learning problem, it is evident that an interrelationship among the classroom teacher, the resource room teacher, and the speech–language clinician is mandatory if suitable services are to be provided for such children. The speech–language clinician frequently assumes a leadership position in the M-Team deliberations and the subsequent individual educational program (IEP) designed for children with educational problems as well as communicative disorders. The objective of the M-Team is to share information describing the nature and dynamics of the learning disorder(s) and speech–language problem(s) and to design an appropriate academic and treatment environment for the child.

Other members of the M-Team may be a psychologist, an educational specialist, the school principal, counselor, social worker, and other specialists as well as the aforementioned regular and/or special education (resource room) teacher. It is assumed that if the child possesses a communication disorder, the team will include a speech–language clinician.

A free and open discussion of the child's multifaceted problems by all members of the team—including, of course, the teacher and parent—should be conducted. Yet, in some schools such discussions are relatively rare. Also, one member of the team may dominate the interaction among team members so that an almost dictatorial atmosphere is generated; in such cases, the teacher and/or parent frequently are unable to participate meaningfully in the discussion. Needless to say, such nonparticipation on the part of the team members handicaps, perhaps very significantly, the planning of an appropriate program design for the child. Furthermore, the lack of opportunity for candid interactions does not permit the teacher and/or parent to participate fully in the education–habilitation of the child. All members of the team should therefore be encouraged to actively participate and voice their agreement or disagreement with the specialists who present their test results.

The very nature of the test situation often prevents positive test results. Test scores that are not reliable are of limited value—indeed, they may even be harmful since learning and treatment programs are designed from the results of test scores. If the teacher or parent does not believe the score appropriately "pictures" the child's problems, these reservations should be stated.

If the mutual decision of the M-Team is to place the child in the regular classroom and the resource room, it is immediately apparent that the conventional classroom teacher must understand the nature of the child's problem(s) and exactly what has to be done to help the child in the classroom. Unfortunately, such knowledge is not always possessed or transmitted to the classroom teacher. As a consequence, the teacher frequently harbors much anxiety about such classroom placement. If mainstreaming is not as effective as it could be, it may be due, in part, to the lack of teacher understanding regarding the communicatively impaired and exceptional child.

6

How Children Acquire Language: Auditory Processing Skills and their Importance in K-2

Sol Adler

The acquisition of acceptable oral language requires the possession of unimpaired auditory processing behaviors. Such behaviors are not only foundational to normal speech–language development but also are related to the development of satisfactory reading and writing skills.

Thus, children not only must hear a verbal stimulus but also must attend to, retain, recognize, and discriminate it, sequence the discrete sounds in the message, and finally, conceptualize and understand it. All of these latter functions are currently termed *auditory processing*. Similar activities likewise occur in the brain with other sensory stimuli such as visual, touch, feel, and smell. At some point in time all of these experiences are integrated into a whole, and the child has complete knowledge of the stimulus. Teachers must recognize that children who possess a deficiency in oral language, reading, or writing, may also possess a disorder in their auditory acuity and processing skills.

AUDITORY ATTENTION

Children who are easily distracted, who do not pay appropriate attention to you when you are teaching, possess what is termed an *attention deficit disorder* (ADD). A clear relationship exists between ADD and behavior disorders. Children who are hyperactive and/or easily distracted will have severely limited auditory attention

ORAL COMMUNICATION PROBLEMS
IN CHILDREN AND ADOLESCENTS
Copyright © 1988 by Grune & Stratton, Inc.

ISBN 0-8089-1887-7
All rights reserved.

spans. These youngsters may possess great academic potential but will be unable to utilize it if they cannot pay appropriate attention. Such children should receive intensive behavior management training, when possible, by a school psychologist.*

At the beginning of the year, approximately half the children in kindergarten manifest ADD. They have poor selective attention; that is, they are easily distracted by random or background noises and have difficulty therefore focusing on what you may be saying. As the children mature, the number of children who manifest ADD decreases in the first grade to approximately a quarter to a third (e.g., one might expect that in a class of 25 first graders, some 6 to 8 of the children exhibit ADD), and in the second grade, to one or two such children. In K-2 these behaviors usually are normal and may be related to maturational lags (i.e., the "late bloomers"); however, the earlier children manifest acceptable selective attention, the better their learning behavior in the classroom. Conversely, the later the appearance of appropriate selective attention, the poorer their learning behavior. Much can be done to enhance such behavior during the preschool years through "figure-ground" training concepts. That is, children who seem to have problems in attending to a selected stimulus—who are easily distracted—can be taught to pay attention to the desired stimulus by increasing its loudness level (or size if it is a visual stimulus) and decreasing background noises.

Children who manifest such difficulties should not be placed in the "open" classroom; they need a structured setting. Furthermore, kindergarten children with ADD probably should not be promoted to the first grade but rather to a higher level of kindergarten (or perhaps they should be held back in the same class), until an acceptable level of selective attention is demonstrated.

Also, children manifesting poor selective attention in the third grade or beyond probably possess a pathologic condition causing the disorder and will need remedial help. They might even benefit from psychopharmacologic agents—drugs—such as Ritalin (CIBA, Summit, NJ) to help control the behavior problems and thereby enhance the selective attention.

It is of interest to note that all preschool-age children possess random rather than selective attention. For some reason (perhaps early maturation and/or training), a number of children develop good selective attention earlier in life than others; theses are the children who can profit significantly from early placement in the academic classroom. The late bloomers or children, who develop such ability later in life but who are placed in an academic setting before they are maturationally ready, become easily frustrated and often develop a personality pattern inappropriate to acceptable learning behavior.

---

* Nutritional disorders may cause some children to manifest ADD. Allergies, too much sugar, inappropriate or absent meals may cause behavior problems and thus ADD. We once recommended to a kindergarten teacher to give white milk or an apple to each child in her class soon after the school day began. The results were very encouraging.

AUDITORY RETENTION

When a teacher gives a two- or three-part command to the children in the classroom, it is expected that they all can (1) hear it, ((2) attend to it, and (3) retain it in order for them to perform adequately what the teacher has asked of them. Some children in K-2, however, possess problems in (1), (2), or (3) above. All children who perform inadequately on a test preceded by a number of directions should be examined to see if, in fact, they heard, attended to, and retained the test directions.

A simple test that can be used to ascertain whether or not such children have adequate short-term memory for the directions is the *Oral Comprehension Sub-Test of the Detroit Test of Learning Aptitudes*. It is a simple test and should be administered to all children with learning and/or behavioral problems.

Children who perform poorly on such tests are not going to be good test takers or will perform generally at their potential. The Oral-Commissions test can be used as a rapid screening tool to identify those students who are high-risk for such activities.

RECOGNITION AND DISCRIMINATION

Children must learn to perceive auditory stimuli—sounds and words—under listening conditions that may make such discrimination difficult. Figure-ground difficulties or background discrimination problems can be tested by the speech–language pathologist.

SEQUENCING

Related terms are phonics, phonemic synthesis, and auditory blending. In essence, all pertain to the child's ability to integrate properly the sounds in a word so that the correct word is heard and can be said by the child.† This auditory sequencing skill, according to some researchers, is of much importance. Disordered sequential skills may cause articulation, reading, and spelling disorders. Children possessing any one or more of these disorders should be tested for their auditory sequencing abilities.

CONCEPT-FORMATION AND AURAL LANGUAGE

The last "event" in this auditory processing chain allows the verbal stimulus to be appropriately categorized and/or classified (i.e., concept–formation) and finally

---

† Or conversely, to break down a word into its component sounds, a task requiring analysis skills.

understood. If children have difficulty with their concept–formation skills, their judgmental abilities may be impaired, or they may have trouble associating a word with the proper referent. For example, the word *ring* may pertain to what is worn on a finger as the term is used in a sentence; yet children may have trouble with the abstraction involved and think that *ring* relates to a telephone ringing. Thus, their response to the sentence will be unusual.

PART II

The Disorders

7

A Brief Introduction to the Disorders

Sol Adler

INTRODUCTION TO LANGUAGE DEFICIENCIES

Causes

Children whose inability to understand and/or speak properly words and/or sentences possess disorders that are obviously detrimental to school learning. Whether the cause is due to some failure or inadequacy in the child's environment, hearing impairment, brain dysfunction, genetic disorder, or biochemical malfunction, the resultant language disorder may range from mild disturbance to severe disability.

Inadequate language environment. An inadequate language environment is due to a paucity of appropriate linguistic stimulation whereby the parents or caretakers rarely provide a need for intelligible and appropriate language usage.

Hearing impairment. An inability to hear correctly what is being said usually will cause an expressive language disorder. Thus children with mild-moderate-severe hearing losses will commonly manifest inappropriate oral language patterns.

Brain dysfunction. Brain dysfunction is due to a variety of causes, for example, brain damage, heredity, food allergies, etc., the child may manifest mild-moderate-severe language–learning problems as well as academic-learning disorders, behavior disorders, etc. If the dysfunction is sufficiently severe it may cause mental retardation.

Genetic disorder. Genetic disorders may be inherited or caused by genetic impairments such as excess radiation, maternal age, or biochemical pollution. Resul-

ORAL COMMUNICATION PROBLEMS
IN CHILDREN AND ADOLESCENTS
Copyright © 1988 by Grune & Stratton, Inc.
ISBN 0-8089-1887-7

tant abnormal chromosomes or inborn error of metabolism affects the child's mentality—the ability to learn appropriate language symbols.

Biochemical malfunction. A malfunctioning biochemical system can cause a variety of different problems. For example, childhood autism and the unusual use of language is suspected of being related to such a cause. Or, some brain dysfunction may result from the impaired chemical functioning and in turn result in a specific language disturbance.

Treatment

To appropriately treat and educate such children requires: (1) an effective interaction among the teacher, parent, and speech–language pathologist; (2) a determination of the cause of the problem; and (3) an intensive remedial program.

INTRODUCTION TO LANGUAGE DIFFERENCES

Children from the lower classes who are both economically disadvantaged and culturally different, frequently speak in a nonstandard dialect. These dialectal patterns, different from standard English, are, in fact, rule-governed and appropriate linguistic and paralinguistic patterns (i.e., body language and speech prosody).

Conventional wisdom in the public schools often dictates that such speech–language usage is substandard and incorrect, and must be eradicated. Few school systems, however, succeed in teaching a majority of these children to speak in standard English.

Due to the children's inability to speak competently in standard English, they generally manifest much difficulty in learning to read and write in standard English. Many of the culturally different and poor children in this country fall behind significantly in their reading levels, as well as other academic skills, due in part to the linguistc and cultural conflicts that exist in the typical classroom.

There are three intervention approaches to the following social dialect patterns—black English, appalachian English, and hispanic English: (1) The eradication of the dialects with the assumption that they are substandard and incorrect speech utterances. This strategy has not worked efficiently; most social dialect speakers retain their cultural-social speech behaviors. (2) The acceptance of the dialects with the assumption that they are rule-governed, that it is part of the cultural heritage, and therefore there is no legitimate reason to do anything about the dialectal patterns. (3) The bidialectal approach that accepts the legitimacy of the social dialect, but realizes that it penalizes its user in both education and employment opportunities. This teaching strategy involves the utilization of an "everyday or home dialect" and a "school dialect," with the child learning to switch dialectal usage according to the situation.

INTRODUCTION TO VOICE DISORDERS

Both elementary-age and adolescent-age children and teenagers may manifest a variety of voice problems: (1) *pitch*—too high or too low for their age, sex, and/or stature; (2) *loudness*—too loud or too soft for the classroom environment; (3) *quality*—either nasality problems characterized by too much (hypernasality—"talking through the nose") or too little (hyponasality—similar to the sound of the voice when one has a head cold) nasality; or chronic hoarse or husky voice quality resulting from inappropriate pitch or loudness usage, or by some organic pathology. Inappropriate usage of the vocal mechanism is quite common and requires vocal re-education by a trained speech–language pathologist, while the various pathologies that can result in chronic hoarseness require the services of a laryngologist.

In vocal re-education, once the correct level of pitch has been ascertained by the speech–language pathologist, the child must remember to talk with the "new voice." This is difficult for the child to monitor and requires the help of the adults who interact with the child. As with articulation disorders, it is desirable that a "carryover" technique be administered by the teacher that will help the child re-member to use the correct voice in the classroom.

A teacher should be able to identify voice disorders in children and adolescents. Yet classroom teacher accuracy in identifying these disorders is very low. Teachers (and parents) often overlook voice problems.

A variety of surveys, regarding the incidence of these disorders, shows that approximately 6 percent of school-age children possess voice problems but that only about 10 percent of these children are recognized by the teachers.

Clearly, a systematic in-service training program by the speech–language pathologist that provides the teachers with recognition criteria would be most useful. For example, such programs entailing (1) an explanation of vocal abuse and misuse, and (2) the different voice disorders, as well as (3) the relevant anatomic features, have proven to be very successful.

INTRODUCTION TO STUTTERING

Stuttering has an ancient heritage. It was recorded in the writings of the ancient Greeks and Egyptians. In the Old Testament it is said that Moses "was slow of tongue" (it is generally accepted that this is a reference to stuttering). This should not be surprising; many prominent historical figures have been stutterers.

An insidious disease, stuttering (or its synonym stammering) usually starts during preschool years and increases in severity as the child progresses from child-hood to adolescence to adulthood. Stuttering is insidious because people are simply unaware of the magnitude of its effect upon the stutterer. The concordance between the abnormal repetitions and prolongations that typify this oral abnormality, and the high anxiety and fear levels manifested by stutterers frequently make their lives a chronically unhappy one for them.

Anxiety and fear are generated by society's disapproval of stuttering: people tend to be impatient with stuttering behavior and may manifest this impatience in ways that are psychologically harmful to the stutterer. For example, children or adolescents who are responding to a teacher's question, and stutter as they do so, may experience peer laughter, or a teacher may give them unsatisfactory advice on how to "cure themselves."

Younger stutterers have little awareness or anxiety regarding their dysfluency pattern; as they become older and receive negative reactions to their stuttering, they learn to fear stuttering. They try to avoid stuttering by learning to utilize "tricks" in their attempt not to stutter when they talk. Unfortunately, these tricks that are of some help initially, soon become automatic behavior and no longer give them the desired fluency. Now they not only stutter but the stuttering may be accompanied by relatively bizarre behaviors, for example, blinking or shutting the eyes, moving an arm and/or leg, facial grimace, and so on. Therefore, the prognosis for cure is best during the preschool years or early school years; however, it should be noted that the pressures and tensions inherent in school detract from the possibility of a cure.

The secondary stutterer usually is taught to live with the problem; to try to become objective about it; to cope with the varied problems caused by the disorder; and to eliminate some of the fear and anxiety mentioned above. With the attenuation of this covert psychological problem there is generally a significant decrease in overt stuttering.

There are those, generally nonqualified practitioners, who claim to be able to cure the disorder in children and adolescents. Conversely, there are qualified clinicians experimenting with newer therapeutic approaches. The teacher or parent must carefully evaluate the credentials of these people.

INTRODUCTION TO ARTICULATION DISORDERS

There are four different kinds of articulation deficiencies: (1) omissions, for example, -oup instead of soup, sou- for soup; (2) additions, for example, idea*r* instead of idea, statistic*s* for statistic; (3) distortions, for example, an utterance not quite appropriate, lateral lisps, trilled "r"; and (4) substitutions, for example, Ru*p* instead of Ruth, free for tree. The first and last patterns—omissions and substitutions—are the most common mistakes made by children. Articulatory disorders account for approximately three-quarters to four-fifths of caseloads for speech-language pathologists in the public schools; there is little question that the classroom teacher and parent (or caregiver) can do much to enhance the child's articulatory skills, and thereby help eliminate the problem.

Many of these articulation problems stem from (1) poor speech models and (2) insufficient and/or inappropriate stimulation.* Clearly, these causes of articulation disorders are the most prevalent and can be obviated through teacher–parent cooperation with the speech–language pathologist. Whenever a child says something that is articulated incorrectly, the listener should be taught to (1) correct overtly by saying to the child, "Johnny, the correct way to say the word is ____," or (2) correct covertly by repeating what the child just uttered—but saying it correctly while emphasizing the target sound in the target word. Other causes of articulatory disturbances will require the skilled attention of the speech–language pathologist, but the teacher also can be of much help. For example, in traditional articulation therapy programs children can be taught to say the sound correctly within the confines of the therapy room, but may have much difficulty in remembering to say it correctly out of the therapy room in conventional "everyday" interactions with people, particularly in the classroom. By alerting a given child to the need to "remember," the teacher can enhance this "carryover" process from therapy room to classroom. This alerting process can be accomplished by some code that has been pre-arranged between the teacher and child, for example, a pull on the ear lobe whenever the child is about to speak in the classroom.

INTRODUCTION TO HEARING PROBLEMS

An increasing number of hearing-impaired children are being placed in regular classrooms or in special classes in public schools. This increase is due in large measure to PL 94-142 (see p 4) and its provision of a least-restrictive class placement (or environment) for handicapped children. As a consequence of this placement, teachers are now compelled to understand and deal effectively with these children.

A recent survey† indicated a lack of understanding of hearing loss and its implications by both regular classroom teachers, and special education or special class teachers. As a result, it was suggested that the following items be included in

---

* Both of these causes are frequently interrelated. The former pertains to a person—parent, relative, teacher, sibling, friend—who possesses an articulation disorder and because of a modeling effect encourages the child to manifest a similar disorder. The latter pertains generally to a family constellation in which there is a lack of concern regarding correct articulation, for example, the substandard articulation manifested by the child is acceptable to the parents who do not correct the child's deficient utterance(s). In such circumstances there is little need for good speech behavior.

It should be noted that the speech–language pathologist can accomplish little with children whose defective articulation stems from such etiologies unless the environmental causes as noted above can be altered. If classroom teachers would use their influence, in conjunction with the efforts of the speech–language pathologist to persuade the models to make appropriate changes in their speech behavior, much good could be accomplished.

† See NJ Lass, et al. *A Survey of Classroom Teachers* and Special Educators *Knowledge of and Exposure to Hearing Loss, LSHSS,* July, 1985.

continuing education programs for teachers and special educators. These items have formed the core for the chapters dealing with this problem:

1. prevalence, etiology, types, and severity of hearing loss
2. assessment of hearing loss in children of different ages
3. procedures for identifying children in school, who should be referred for hearing screening
4. receptive and expressive communication problems of hearing-impaired children and implications for their learning in the classroom
5. medical and nonmedical treatment of hearing loss
6. medical and nonmedical professionals who work with hearing-impaired children
7. general principles of aural rehabilitation
8. manual communication and its application to hearing-impaired children
9. general structure and function of hearing aids and their use with hearing-impaired children.

Children with mild to moderate hearing disorders may attend the regular classroom; and those with more severe hearing problems may also participate in the normal classroom but will need an interpreter. The mild problems some children manifest frequently go undetected by the classroom teacher or parents. For example, during the winter months there is often an increase in hearing problems due to colds, yet these problems are often not recognized by the teacher. If such problems persist, that is, become chronic, they may cause substantial learning disorders in the child. Mild hearing problems, when accompanied by pain or a foul smelling discharge from the ears, are instantly recognizable, but the mere presence of the mild hearing loss in itself may not alert the teacher or parent to the existence of such a problem. The only alerting signal may be a change in the behavioral status of the child. A visit to the otologist generally treats such a problem very effectively.

Moderate hearing problems are noticeable and require special care: amplification and auditory training procedures. The former pertains to hearing aid usage, the latter to teaching children to make optimum use of their residual hearing—perhaps including speech reading (synonymous to lip reading) and special seating arrangements. Teachers must be aware that a child utilizing a hearing aid has to become acclimated to the amplification offered by the aid and that this requires a period of training. The child with a more severe hearing problem, who is not attending a school for the deaf, may be integrated into the conventional classroom for a part or all of the school day, and may require the services of an interpreter.

8

Language Deficiencies

Jane E. Robinson
Asa J. Brown

If you desire ease, forsake learning.
If you desire learning, forsake ease.
How can the man at his ease acquire knowledge,
And how can the earnest student enjoy ease?

From: Aphorisms
The Tree of Wisdom
(Tibetan Buddhist literature)

EDITOR'S INTRODUCTION

The nature of language deficiencies in children and what the teacher can do to help such children acquire improved language skills are explained in some detail. Aural-oral language is of basic importance to the acquisition of academic skills; children manifesting an impaired ability to understand and/or use appropriate linguistic symbols in their verbal communications frequently will manifest significant problems in their academic classwork.

Drs. Robinson and Brown have worked closely with teachers for many years; they are familiar with their problems and address their needs in a very concrete manner in this chapter.

LANGUAGE LEARNING—BIRTH THROUGH HIGH SCHOOL

Language learning in normal children happens almost like magic. There is a natural progression from the reflexive cries of a newborn, to the emergence of the first words and phrases of 1- and 2-year-olds, to the use of many adult grammatical forms by 4- and 5-year-olds. During this progression normal infants, toddlers, and preschoolers acquire not only the content and form of their native language, but also

ORAL COMMUNICATION PROBLEMS
IN CHILDREN AND ADOLESCENTS
Copyright © 1988 by Grune & Stratton, Inc.

ISBN 0-8089-1887-7
All rights reserved.

many of the communicative variations necessary for increasing conversational sophistication.

As children enter their formal school years, they continue to expand their oral language skills, especially in the areas of vocabulary and conversational abilities. These oral communication skills are prerequisites for academic success. Effective oral communication is the basis for the acquisition of higher level reading and writing skills. While the focus on basic skills tends to emphasize reading and writing during the elementary years, there is a high expectation of age-level oral communication in the middle and high school years (i.e., note-taking abilities in content area courses).

LANGUAGE AND EDUCATIONAL SUCCESS

Normal language acquisition perplexes us as professionals faced with the obligation of educating language-impaired students. If normal language is acquired with such apparent ease, then how can we as educators encourage and enhance language development in our students? How can we remediate language disorders in our language-impaired students? It is acceptable to be bewildered as a novice; it is less acceptable to remain so.

Educators must sacrifice the desire for ease and demand information that is current, theoretically based, and applicable in their classrooms. It is with this thought in mind that we attempt to make this chapter accurate not only in content and form, but also useful to you as educators. It is because we are all confronted with the communicative struggles, both academic and social, of language-impaired students that we will mutually forsake our ease and investigate aspects of language learning in this special population.

LANGUAGE DEFICIENCIES*

Language deficiencies are nondiscriminatory. Both regular education and special education classrooms are the home-base for language-impaired students. Language deficiencies occur across the wide age-range of public school students. In the regular education setting, this range spans the years from preschool throughout high school. Special education populations encompass a wider age-span, with eligible students aged 3–21 receiving service as a result of PL 94-142 (see p 4 for definition). Increasingly, there is also a national trend to provide service to infants who are considered to be at-risk for language handicaps from birth. Because oral language is the basis for academic achievement, it is no wonder that we must prioritize our responsibility to learn more about the process of human communication.

---

*Language deficiencies, as used here, includes many terms that are frequently used in various texts and in various states. It is used generically to mean either delayed or deviant language behaviors. These terms are explained later in the chapter.

CHAPTER OBJECTIVES

Our major objective in this chapter is to assist you, the educator, as you sort out the perplexities of oral language deficiencies and place them into a workable instructional perspective. As you progress through this chapter, keep in mind that deficient oral language is the single most significant deterrent to educational growth.

This chapter is not directed at a specific age-level or any specific type of language deficiency. We urge you to take the practical knowledge of your language arts teaching background and broaden it. Although some of you may have special interests in specific areas of special education, remember that both budget and programming problems could result in an unsolicited transfer across age-levels or job descriptions (i.e., from a preschool learning disabilities classroom to a resource room in a high school setting).

High-incidence populations. In an attempt to meet the needs of the majority of our readers, we have narrowed the immediate focus to high-incidence special populations; that is, language-impaired students in regular education classes, learning disabilities classes, educable mentally impaired classes, and emotionally impaired classes. The group of students listed above includes those language-impaired students whom we expect to be academically successful. This group of students contrasts with those in low-incidence populations, including those special students who are more severely impaired (i.e., autistic, severely mentally impaired, multiply-impaired).

One subgroup of language-deficient students is not eligible for special education services. Their difficulties with oral language are not substantial enough to meet state and federal criteria for special education placement, including speech/language services. They will, however, be enrolled in your classes! These marginal communicators (Blue, 1975) depend on the expertise of regular educators for three extremely important reasons:

1. They are at-risk for academic and social failure.
2. True language deficiencies may surface as these students increase in age because of ever increasing classroom performance expectations.
3. You, as their teachers, may be the only professionals to suspect emerging oral language deficiencies.

Specific Objectives

The remainder of the chapter is designed to help you decrease your perplexities about educating language-deficient students. Specifically, we anticipate that our readers will

1. increase their understanding of normal language and its development (see the Appendix);

2. increase their understanding of the nature of language deficiencies;
3. increase their understanding of team approaches for identifying language- deficient students;
4. increase their understanding of both the *academic* and *social* significance of appropriate oral language programming in the classroom.

Our focus is on school-age students. We are addressing students whom we expect to succeed both academically and socially. Educational success and effective oral communication skills are inseparable. We urge you to also expect success—both academic and social—from this very special group of students.

LANGUAGE DEFICIENCIES

Definitions

Language disorders, which may be broken up into the categories of language delay and language deviance, are defined as follows.

Language disorders. A current definition of language disorders, drafted by the Committee on Language, Speech, and Hearing Services in the Schools of the American Speech–Language–Hearing Association (ASHA, 1982), is

A language disorder is the impairment or deviant development of comprehension and/ or use of a spoken, written, and/or other symbol system. This disorder may involve (1) the form of language (phonologic, morphologic, and syntactic systems), (2) the content of language (semantic system) and/or (3) the function of language in communication (pragmatic system) in any combination. (*24*, pp 949–950)

Consequently, we view a language disorder as the inability of an individual to understand and/or use the language systems of society. Such a disorder may range from a minor developmental delay in the acquisition of language to the complete absence of the ability to use language for communication (ASHA, 1982, pp 949–950).

Language delay/language deviance. Sometimes language disorders are divided into two separate categories. The first, *language delay*, usually refers to marked slowness in the development of language. The second, *deviant language*, customarily refers to language development that does not synchronize with or parallel the expected age-related stages. Within the present focus on the high-incidence populations, the differentiation is not emphasized. Rather, both delayed and deviant language are included within the more generic label of *language deficiencies*. Also included in the more general category of language deficiencies is that group of students who have language delays that are not significant enough to warrant special education intervention (i.e., the marginal communicators).

In Bloom and Lahey's (1978) model, the representation of *form, content,* and *use* implies an overlapping development of all the parameters of language. This is widely accepted when describing normal language acquisition. However, when children and/or adolescents do not acquire normal language skills, there may be a distortion of the relationship between the three portions of the language system named above.

Language Deficiencies in Various High-Incidence Populations

Within the high-incidence population of language-impaired students considered in this chapter, we might alter Bloom and Lahey's representations of *form, content* and *use*. With educable mentally impaired students, each portion would approach, but not quite reach, normal expectations. Thus, an educable youngster might have a limited vocabulary, use simple concrete grammatical structures, and not acquire all of the conversational complexities of their normal peers. Emotionally impaired youngsters might have intact grammatical systems, but distortions in the semantic (meaning) system as it relates to judgment and higher level functions. There would be a resultant reduction in the use of language for interpersonal communication. Learning-disabled youngsters may have impairments in all areas, but they would not necessarily be as easily categorized as those of a youngster with cognitive deficits (i.e., the educable student).

Regular education students with language impairments may fit into any of the above personal profiles, although they may lack definitive diagnostic criteria for specific special education eligibility; that is, they remain in the regular education setting. Those who are eligible receive speech and language services; those who are mildly impaired may not receive any special education services.

Language Deficiencies and Listening Skills

The definition of language deficiencies used here is more global and all encompassing than many traditional definitions. It is based upon the assumption that language and communication are a synergistic system—a *process* (Prutting, 1979). Further, our definition and perspective assumes that

> . . . language disabilities can no longer be viewed only as receptive-expressive break-downs. Likewise, such skills as auditory discrimination, auditory sequential memory, and the like need to be interpreted within the context of what we know about language and communication systems. Memory is more than memory for sequences of digits . . . (AHSA, 1982, pp 940–941)

Specific Language Behaviors

The literature pertaining to language disorders in the school-age population frequently differentiates between language behaviors (those directly related to the five parameters of language) and more general behaviors commonly identified in language-impaired students. Examples of specific language behaviors include the following:

1. reduced vocabulary
2. restricted sentence length
3. omission of morphological markers such as plurals and tense markers†
4. omission of or limited use of modifiers, articles, and/or prepositions
5. restricted ability to use language for giving and receiving interpersonal information

General Listening Skills

The specific language behaviors listed above can be contrasted with more general behavior characteristics that interfere with language acquisition and language use. The general behaviors include a collection of factors commonly referred to as listening skills, auditory processing, or information processing factors. As a group these factors are closely related to specific learning expectations in the classroom. Examples of these general behaviors are:

1. attention to tasks and to classroom instructions/discussion
2. memory for series of instructions/explanations
3. organizational skills (i.e., ability to sort out important information from the massive amounts of verbal input in the classroom)
4. evaluative skills (i.e., ability to make judgments about the relevance and truth of classroom lectures/discussions)

According to Johnson and Myklebust (1967), many students are limited in the amount of information they can remember. Such students will experience difficulty in the classroom because in order to comprehend complex verbal instructions, they must first be able to "take in" a series of connected sentences. As Johnson and Myklebust (1967) aptly pointed out, problems with *memory* are differentiated from specific language deficiencies.

> A language impaired student may be unable to follow a command because he does not understand the *words* or word combinations. . . . A student with a limited memory span understands the words and the single series of words in a command but has difficulty retaining a series of sentences. (p 111)

This distinction becomes primary to our increased understanding of language-impaired students. We should be able to distinguish between those students who have difficulty with spoken language due to impairments in any of the five parameters and those students who have difficulty processing information received through auditory input due to deficient listening skills. Listening is not only relevant in the classroom, but also a requisite for vocational/employment success.

---

†In the following chapter by Dr. Bountress it is noted that some of these behaviors are related to one's dialect community and hence are not substandard but rather nonstandard utterances.

Language and Listening as a Function of Age

Recent literature again focuses on listening, as it relates to language skills in older students (Boyce & Lord-Larson, 1983; Butler, 1984; Simon, 1985; Wiig, 1984). As students approach the middle school years, the verbal demands increase both in academic and social terms. In a recent position paper addressing language learning disabilities, ASHA (1982) proposed that language-deficient children

> . . . don't necessarily catch up. The early forms of language disorders are seen as varying problems in the comprehension and/or use of language symbols as well as disturbances in the social use of language. In addition, many of these children present deficits in their ability to use and organize incoming auditory information. (*24*, p 938)

This point is also dramatically apparent in a follow-up study of language-impaired preschoolers reported by Aram, Ekelman, and Nation (1984). They concluded that children with language disorders during their preprimary years do not present disorders confined only to spoken language. The majority of the subjects presented broadly based language–learning, educational, and social problems throughout their school years. Within the school setting, the language arts curriculum is typically divided into age-related categories. The basic categories include preprimary, primary, later elementary, and middle/high school. The present focus emphasizes not only those categories but the transitions between them. It is possible that many language-deficient students at-risk for academic/social failure surface at the transition points.

Summary of Definition of Language Deficiencies

The following list summarizes the definition of language deficiencies:

1. Language deficiencies include both developmental delays and deviant development in the understanding and/or use of language for communication.
2. Language deficiencies involve the form, content, and use of language.
3. While listening and processing skills are intricately related to language ability, they can be distinguished in important ways.
4. Language deficiencies have many common characteristics across high-incidence special education categories (i.e., emotional impairments, learning disabilities, educable mentally impaired).
5. Some language-deficient students are not sufficiently impaired to meet state/federal guidelines for special education services.
6. There are important age-related differences in the characteristics of language-deficient students.

IDENTIFYING LANGUAGE-IMPAIRED STUDENTS

In the public school setting, the system used for the identification of language-deficient students who are eligible for special education services is a *process*. The

Individualized Educational Planning Committee (IEPC) is comprised of a group of professionals concerned with assessment, eligibility, and programming. The assessment team, called the Multidisciplinary Team (M-Team) minimally consists of a certified speech–language pathologist and the classroom teacher. Input is also solicited from the parent and the student, when appropriate. The IEPC process for identifying and planning intervention for language-deficient students is explained in the following section.

The IEPC Process

The M-Team, as established by PL 94-142, is paramount as a vehicle for accomplishing the task of identifying and determining intervention goals for language-impaired students. There is a logical progression of transdisciplinary procedures that begins with the referral of students suspected of being language-impaired. Assessment of oral language skills is the next step, followed by the determination of eligibility for speech and language services. As the process is completed, language goals and objectives are formulated and implemented through the cooperative efforts of the classroom teacher and the speech–language pathologist. The involvement of the classroom teacher is mandated by PL 94-142 throughout this entire process.

Referral

Listen to your students! The classroom teacher is the most common referral source for language-impaired students. Damico and Oller, Jr. (1980) reported that teachers are usually expected to refer students based on "surface form" criteria. These criteria are aspects of the grammatical system, such as correct tenses, pronouns, etc. However, pragmatic criteria, related to the student's ability to use language for giving and receiving information, seemed to be superior for identifying language-disordered students. The differentiation between grammatical-structural criteria and pragmatic criteria is particularly relevant as we consider the differences in our expectations for normal language competencies across the school ages of 3–21. Table 8-1 illustrates some examples of the various criteria used by classroom teachers as they listen to their students.

Assessment

The sole professional mandated to diagnose *oral* language impairments is the person certified to do so—the speech–language pathologist. The certified speech–language pathologist is the professional who administers and interprets formal language tests. The formal language assessment usually includes an analysis of a spontaneous language sample. The classroom teacher is required to provide input during the assessment procedures. This equally important role involves the provision of

Table 8-1
Comparison of Grammatical vs. Pragmatic Referral Criteria

Grammatical Criteria	Pragmatic Criteria
1. Noun–verb agreement *The cat run* vs. *The cat runs*	1. Linguistic nonfluency Speech production contains a high incidence of unusual pauses, repetitions, and/or hesitations.
2. Possessive inflections *Linda book* vs. *Linda's book*	2. Revisions Speech production contains a high incidence of false starts or self-interruptions.
3. Verb tenses *The cat run* vs. *The cat is running*	3. Delays before responding Attempts at speech production in response to questions or requests from others are delayed by long pauses.
4. Irregular verbs *The cat eated* vs. *The cat ate*	4. Nonspecific vocabulary Excessive use of *this, that* without reference along with excessive use of generic terms such as *thing* and *stuff.*
5. Irregular plurals *The sheeps ate* vs. *The sheep ate*	5. Inappropriate responses Responses or narratives that proceed without reference to the listener.
6. Pronoun case or gender *Linda brought him book* vs. *Linda brought her book*	6. Poor topic maintenance Rapid and inappropriate changes in the topic without providing transitional clues to the listener.
7. Syntactic transpositions *The book blue is on the table* vs. *The blue book is on the table*	7. Need for repetition Multiple repetitions by the student do not lead to increased comprehension by the listener.

Source: Adapted from Damico J, & Oller Jr JW (1980). Pragmatic versus morphological/syntactic criteria for language referrals. *Language, Speech and Hearing Services in Schools, 11,* 88.

accurate, ongoing descriptions of the communicative effectiveness of students in a variety of school settings.

Descriptions of communicative behavior provided by the classroom teacher should be as specific as possible. Knowledge of normal language development and the referral criteria in Table 8-1 are both necessary aids for this task. Depending on the communicative abilities of particular students, teachers may be forced to make inferences as they provide descriptions of oral communication. If it is necessary to make inferences, then situational cues should be included to reduce the ambiguity of assumptions about the student's intent. The descriptions provided by the classroom teacher might include:

1. examples of oral communication difficulties in the classroom
2. examples of how these specific difficulties have had an adverse effect on educational performance or social adjustment

As a caution to all of us, let us keep in mind two important issues. First, as addressed by Bountress in his chapter on cultural language differences (see Chapter 9), we must sort out those aspects of oral language that are nonstandard from those that are deficiencies in a developing language system. Second, Naremore and Hipskind (1979) strikingly demonstrated that professionals (speech–language pathologists in training) heard grammatical errors that *were not present* when told they were listening to language samples of educable mentally impaired students. Think about the impact this has on our objectivity as listeners, especially for those of us who are special educators. If we unconsciously have stereotypes of the linguistic abilities of various groups of special students, we may unassumingly bias our descriptive judgments of their performance.

Placement

The IEPC includes a minimum of one member of the M-Team, who presents the team recommendations; a school administrator; the classroom teacher; the parent; and the student, when appropriate. While the M-Team recommends placement, it is the IEPC that determines eligibility for special education (speech/language) services. Once eligibility has been determined, the IEPC establishes: (1) the amount of time required for appropriate services, (2) individualized annual goals, and (3) short-term instructional objectives.

The IEPC may decide that language goals and objectives will be most appropriately implemented by the speech–language pathologist as a direct service. However, as the concept of "teaming" becomes a reality, more high-incidence language-impaired students will have oral language goals and objectives incorporated into the classroom language arts curriculum. With some of these students, the speech–language pathologist will provide consulting services for a predetermined amount of time. Another option for programming involves the implementation of direct speech/language services within the classroom as opposed to a special speech/language "therapy" room. The group of students who are "borderline" will not be eligible for speech/language services and will depend on the classroom teacher to be sole provider of instruction in oral communication.

ORAL COMMUNICATION IN THE CLASSROOM

Language Arts

The concept of teaming and cooperative programming for language-impaired students is theoretically applicable in all school settings. It is not an unrealistic goal. Classroom teachers and speech–language pathologists can provide shared service! In other sections of this chapter, we defined *normal language*. In terms of shared services, we must also consider the meaning of *language arts*. Is oral language a part of language arts? Is oral language considered to be a basic skill? Is oral language related to literacy?

Academic Language

Typically, the language arts are conceived of as written language, including reading and writing skills. While many language arts curricula include oral language skills during the preschool years, these skills tend to be directed toward teaching vocabulary (generally nouns in categories) and the storytelling activities of the pre-primary years.

As students enter the more formal language arts years, with the development of reading and writing skills, there is a decrease in the amount of time spent on oral communication development in the classroom setting. If oral language is included in the curriculum, it tends to be a group lesson taught as a separate entity at a specifically designated time. Teachers may emphasize general concepts such as the use of complete sentences and "proper" speaking skills. These skills, however, are typically perceived as distinct from reading and writing tasks.

As mentioned previously in the section on language deficiencies, we can divide the aspects of language into three categories: *form*, *content*, and *use*. The major emphasis in language arts is on form (grammatical structures and sentence complexity) and content (especially vocabulary). These aspects of language may be considered a *portion* of the basis for the acquisition of the language of learning. While they are eminently important to the development of language-based academic skills, they frequently are unnecessarily distinguished from the third category—language use.

Interpersonal Language

We, as educators, have long neglected the language of the classroom. We have assumed a common understanding or "mutual intelligibility" (Hymes, 1972, pp xxxvii) between teacher and pupil. According to Hymes, however, a classroom full of students who know the same vocabulary and use the same types of sentences may not have a shared knowledge of the rules for language use (i.e., taking turns; avoiding insults).

Menyuk (1983, p 153) described language development that continues over the school years as focusing on learning a number of higher level communicative variables. Included are such skills as learning how to converse with a teacher and the strategies necessary for argumentation based on hypothetical conditions. These skills are dependent on exposure to the language of the schools.

"The Language of Schooling"

In the academic setting we have traditionally tended to separate language for interpersonal communication from the language of learning. The roles of the speech–language pathologist and the classroom teacher have been dichotomous as a result of this philosophical division. The speech–language pathologist historically has provided direct service to students and emphasized form and content as they relate to interpersonal communication. On the other hand, the classroom teacher has emphasized specific vocabulary (i.e., nouns in categories, shapes, and colors), definitions of words on assigned spelling lists, and the content of texts. Grammatical skills in relation to oral language have been the result of incidental teaching, while the grammar of written language usually has been addressed as a part of isolated "English" assignments. The current cooperative focus involves an overlap between these two previously distinct curricular functions. The speech–language pathologist must address the language of the classroom, both in terms of content and form as related to academics and to the intricate interpersonal aspects of "teacher talk" and "child listening" (Nelson, 1985). Classroom teachers also must shift their focus from the purely academic aspects of the typical language arts curriculum to the broader emphasis on the language of schooling (Butler, 1984; Olson, 1980; Nelson, 1985).

Not all of the language of schooling is verbal, however. Most of the communication carried out in classrooms is a mixture of speech (spoken language) and expressive motor behavior (nonverbal communication). Academic progress is not the only performance area affected by language deficiencies. The entire process of socialization with its heavy dependence on understanding and being understood is also at-risk.

Language Acquisition and Classroom Behavior

Language development and socialization are two interrelated areas of functioning very closely associated with success in school. By the time a youngster reaches school age, however, language deficiencies that were easily observable in their purest form in early childhood tend to become masked. Stevenson, Richman, and Graham (1985) indicate the following with respect to the early presence of language deficiencies and later behavior problems:

> Early language problems are, for some of the children at least, associated with later behavioral deviance, even if later language problems are absent. For this latter group, there is therefore an indication that early remedial language intervention might prevent the development of later behavioral deviance. (p 225)

Because the child must accommodate the increasingly complex social demands of the school environment, over time, deficiencies in language tend to become more and more behaviorally expressed. The degree of impairment will, of course, shape the intensity of the behavioral expression in any given child. The longer children are in school the more they are at-risk that their behavior will be viewed by teachers as a conduct problem and be inappropriately dealt with, albeit with the best of intentions. This situation becomes increasingly evident when youngsters face the dual stressors of adolescence and middle or junior high school.

It may be helpful for classroom teachers to consider the effects of the following three factors when attempting to understand the behavioral manifestations of language deficiency. Common behaviors manifested by language-deficient students are:

1. While the actions of the child may appear at the surface to be purposefully resistive, controlling, or inefficient, the roots of these atypical behaviors often lie in one or more of the deviant language patterns discussed previously. Consulting with a certified speech–language pathologist may be particularly helpful in developing strategies for remediation once specific classroom data have been collected and organized.

2. Language-deficient youngsters go through periods of cognitive disequilibrium when faced with curricular challenges that they are not linguistically prepared to meet. These disequilibrium points are often characterized behaviorally by outbursts of temper, perseveration, or regression. They will be of relatively sudden onset, and upon reflection, can often be associated with the classroom introduction of new and more linguistically demanding material. These reactions tend to cluster at, but are not limited to, certain transition points such as the shift from preschool/kindergarten to first grade, primary to later elementary, and elementary to middle or junior high school. Classroom teachers are encouraged to focus less on the behavioral symptoms of frustration (disequilibrium) shown by the child and more on providing the requisite language competencies needed by the child to successfully manage the new material.

3. The behavior of language-disordered children relates to the classroom management style of the individual teacher. Many of us work in educational settings that tend to stress issues of social conformity and classroom control. This attitude acts to force attention on managing the surface nonconformity of pupils lest the teachers themselves become vulnerable to peer or administrative criticism. This attitude toward socialization and its inherent dangers are well presented by Danziger (1971):

    > Research on socialization has continued to show the influence of what might be called an ideology of social engineering. In reviewing this research it is difficult to escape the impression that much of it has been motivated less by a desire for understanding than by a desire for quick recipes. (pp 14, 17)

    It is important that those working in any educational context *not* fall into the trap of the social engineer. To do so severely limits one's effectiveness by focusing on effect rather than cause and by denying that the socialization process is an interactive one. Language-deficient children by virtue of their unusual and sometimes aberrant behavior certainly affect the socialization mix of the classroom at least as much as they are affected by it.

    A Herculean effort is required to maintain a perspective wherein symptoms are differentiated from causes, an alertness to disequilibrium is maintained, and the interactive nature of socialization is respected. If one is able to accomplish this task, the background is then set for considering some of the common language deficiencies and their behavioral implications.

    For purposes of simplification, we will assume that the language deficiencies of most of the children you will encounter can spring from any of one of three broad conditions: environmental delay, developmental delay, and developmental language disorders. The first condition is the mildest and seems most responsive to normal language enriching strategies (i.e., does not require special education services); the second and third conditions, however, warrant much more intensive intervention by the classroom teacher and the certified speech–language pathologist.

Environmental language delay. Environmental language delay is a term used to describe the most frequent cause of language deficiency—inadequate early language experience. Many youngsters simply do not experience or participate in a sufficiently intense amount of verbal behavior. Their parents and siblings may have engaged in little language conversation; consequently, these young children fail to recognize the social aspects of speech. They are unsure of the potency of language to either produce desired results or form relationships with others. Frequently, this condition is triggered by a lack of richness in language between children and their caregivers. It is not reasonable to infer here that certain cultural situations precondition a child for early language delay, but the work of Bernstein (1971) and others (Randall, Reynell, & Curwen, 1974) has indicated problems do arise when the home language environment is less than favorable for later language use and learning.

The importance of environment in influencing the acquisition of meaning and language in children has received tremendous attention in recent years. Recognition of the importance of early stimulation in this process was one of the prime considerations behind the Head Start movement (initiated in 1965). Unfortunately, as is often the case, many programs and agencies simply proceeded to bombard their charges with verb practice and short cause and effect statements.

Schaffer (1977) summarizes well the feeling of current child development researchers when he remarks that the *amount* of stimulation is not nearly so critical as the *quality* and *style* of stimulation, particularly in the underprivileged:

> . . . 'the more the better' does not do justice to the facts. . . . these children tend to be subjected to a far greater overall level of stimulation: rarely alone, surrounded by a great many adults and endless TV—the total amount of sheer noise impinging on them is likely to be considerable. (pp 57–58)

Quality of environmental stimulation seems to be the more critical factor in comparative research such as that conducted by Kagan and Tulkin (1971). Operationally, this means that parents and teachers should be encouraged to maintain an environment where the child is not just talked to and instructed, but encouraged to take an active participant role. The interactive nature of the socialization process plays an equally important role at home and school. Children are most likely to talk and communicate when persons and events in the environment urge them to so do. A child is much more likely to spontaneously initiate dialogue with an adult if he or she comes from an environment where adults and children interact freely at either person's request. Even in Head Start programs dealing with so-called disadvantaged children there is a tremendous range of language fluency and effectiveness. Most of the more fluent children come from home environments where social interaction is reciprocal.

Respect for the language products of the child is a key factor. The principle is, of course, equally applicable to the classroom. One benchmark as to whether or not the appropriate climate is being maintained is that in the best of circumstances, the child will occasionally interfere with the adult learning agenda.

Developmental language delay. A number of young children have a language delay caused by a constitutional problem rather than external environmental factors. The problem may be mild or severe, depending on the resistance of the child's speech to come forth after intervention. Speech–language pathologists generally consider the difficulty to be a true handicap when the child's receptive and expressive language development is less than two thirds of nonverbal intellectual ability in terms of age. While this is a serious delay and requires close initial intervention, once the child's language does appear it tends to follow a typical pattern of development at least through the stages of early language learning.

Research during the past 20 years has attempted to isolate specific behaviors that surround this dramatically late appearance of language. Most promising among the psychological explanations offered has been the failure of the child's thinking to move from *primary* (action-oriented) to secondary (symbol-oriented) thought processes. Greenacre (1950) and other child psychiatrists (Rexford, 1966) have documented that young children with severe problems of behavioral acting out typically have developmental language delay. Such children's inability to have their strongest needs met through language and symbolic behavior affects their approach to problem solving and conflict resolution. Behaviorally, these children tend to become motoric and are often aggressive.

Lerner, Inui, Trupin, and Douglas (1985) found the following from their longitudinal study of the relationship between preschool behavior and the development of later psychiatric disorders: "Children with speech and language problems had higher rates of psychiatric problems and higher rates of psychiatric disorders than the general population. Children with language delay had a higher prevalence of behavioral disorders" (p 42). Additionally, Gualteri, Koriath, Van Bourgondien, and Saleeby (1983, p 168) found "a strong association, then, between developmental language deficits and severe psychiatric disorders."

The potential for developing behavioral problems is substantially higher for those children with language deficiencies than for those with pure speech difficulties (Baker & Cantwell, 1982; Baker, Cantwell, & Mattison, 1980; Mattison, Cantwell & Baker, 1980). It is important that teachers differentiate between these two groups.

The psychological predisposition for developmental language delay seems to dictate its eventual resolution as well. In most cases, the child's verbal comprehension and expressive language are equally delayed at the onset. But as the youngster grows older, verbal comprehension recovers first, followed by greater fluency in words and sentences, and rounded out eventually by a more mature notion of language "sense" or intelligibility. It should not be forgotten, however, that while this pattern appears to be natural, it is quite late in appearing! Specialized help is required to prevent these youngsters from developing further high-risk language patterns in conjunction with impaired intellectual functioning.

The power of language deficiencies to shape school behavior was dramatically demonstrated by Bloom (1980) in a well controlled study of 60 elementary school children in classrooms for the behaviorally disordered. He found that the incidence of expressive language problems in this population referred and eligible for special education service for treatment of their *deviant behavior* was approximately six times that found in the normal population. He addressed the underlying problem through the use of a simple commercially available language building kit in twice weekly half hour sessions for 18 weeks. The focus was *exclusively* on expressive language development. Bloom found that as expressive language abilities increased, academic performance (reading, spelling, and math) improved; student self-esteem went up; and the level of manifest aggression went down both at the close of the intervention and on 6-month follow-up.

Developmental language disorders.   Certainly the most severe condition for language learning is that of developmental language disorders. In most instances, children with such severe language problems have an additional neurological or intellectual impairment that has caused the linguistic condition. The pattern of such children's language is not only delayed but *deviant;* there is no clear path for development and thus no predictable pattern for recovery. In some children the disorder may be localized on language function (verbal comprehension, for example). Such problems are very difficult to overcome and are never alleviated completely. Many of these children make favorable early progress, but in most cases the development is arrested and language facility reaches a sustained plateau. It is imperative that the teacher work closely with the speech–language pathologist in developing appropriate curricula so that strengths can be capitalized on while remediation is ongoing. This will at least partially reduce the avoidance or aggressive resistance behaviors that characterize many of these children when they are inappropriately challenged.

ISSUES OF INTERVENTION: AN EXPANDED FOCUS

The evidence markedly demonstrates that most language-deficient students do not "catch up" without appropriate intervention throughout their school years. They do, of course, attend school; many of them receive special education services. Traditional services, however, may be too narrow in perspective. One reason for a less than perfect success rate with these students is directly related to the severity of their impairments. Another is the narrow perspective of typical intervention approaches. These approaches have neglected to consider language as a system.

Mutual Intelligibility

The issue of language intervention in the classroom is expertly addressed by Fujiki and Brinton (1984). Their suggestions have consistently piqued the interest of our students in recent years. While acknowledging that the demands of the typical school day leave little time for the teacher to provide individualized instruction, Fujiki and Brinton (pp 98–99) offer many helpful suggestions, of which the major points are listed below:

1. Create a climate of emotional acceptance, emphasizing communication in the classroom.
2. Improve the teacher's listening behavior.
3. Simplify and adjust linguistic input with careful consideration for language complexity.
4. Stress important words.
5. Provide contextual cues (i.e., add extra information to describe and clarify new material).
6. Utilize specific strategies, such as modeling and expanding.
7. Do not ignore unintelligible utterances.

This supports our earlier discussion of Hymes' (1972) concept of mutual intelligibility. In explaining this point, Fujiki and Brinton (1984) reiterate that:

> . . . it is somewhat of a disservice to allow a child to believe that he/she has been understood when he/she has not. . . . Thus, when the teacher does not understand the child, it is the teacher's responsibility to initiate the repair . . . (p 103)

Communication Strategies

We do not communicate in isolated sentences. According to Simon (1985, p 53), prerequisite skills for processing a series of sentences include:

1. the ability to compare new information with old information
2. the ability to evaluate the truth of a message
3. the ability to identify factual errors and absurdities

As students increase in age and grade level, our expectations also increase. Wiig (1984), in an extensive review of the literature pertaining to language intervention, found that: ". . . the most significant implications of the research reviewed appears to be that a shift from teaching specific skills or rules to teaching strategies has to occur to support the attainment of mature language repertoires and communicative competence." (p 53)

These communication strategies involve adaptability on the part of both pupils and teachers! Our emphasis on the oral communication system includes both speaker and listener. In a more general sense we have also emphasized the many motoric or nonverbal aspects of language as they relate to socialization and behavior in the classroom. Just as language-deficient students must learn to identify important points and topics in classroom and personal discussions, we as educators must learn to clarify and organize our messages to these students. We must help them learn to ask for clarification; we must aim to improve their understanding of the *need to understand*. We must encourage their attempts to speak, even though it may sometimes seem time-consuming or disruptive to our own agenda. We must help them also learn the rules of conversation, including when *not* to speak. We must try to develop a sense of inquisitiveness by removing some of the drudgery of structured language drills.

SUMMARY

A central theme throughout this chapter is our belief that "language is both the object of knowledge and the medium through which knowledge is acquired" (Cazden, 1973; also cited in Garrard, 1979, p 92). We have attempted to both persuade you to share our belief and to give you a workable understanding of the nature of language deficiencies. Language-deficient students will benefit from your instruction and personal interaction; mutual intelligibility between teacher and student is a vital and attainable goal.

APPENDIX

Normal Language

In order to understand language impairments, we must first come to some agreement about what normal language is. In normal children we *expect* language to develop! We acknowledge that language is learned in one way or another, but even as naive beginners in the field, we can admit that neither parents nor educators actively set out to *teach* language to normal infants and toddlers. The basic theories underlying the acquisition of language are threefold. First is the behavioristic theory that language is learned as a set of stimulus–response activities. The second basic theory is the nativistic notion that language is prewired in all humans and just as babies learn to walk, they also learn to talk. The environment, of course, must provide exposure to language and children must have the cognitive ability to extract meaning from the sounds, words, and sentences of their environment. The simplest answer to the question of *nature versus nurture* is to accept a third or combination theory. Regardless of the theoretic viewpoint, it is commonly accepted that language is developmental and hierarchical. The building blocks begin in infancy and continue throughout the school years (Menyuk, 1983).

Definition of Language

A current definition of language (ASHA, 1983) states that: Language is a complex and dynamic system of conventional symbols that is used in various modes for thought and communication. Contemporary views of human language hold that

1. language evolves within specific historical, social, and cultural contexts;
2. language as rule-governed behavior is described by at least five parameters—phonologic, morphologic, syntactic, semantic, and pragmatic;
3. language learning and use are determined by the interaction of biological, cognitive, psychosocial, and environmental factors;
4. effective use of language for communication requires a broad understanding of human interaction, including such associated factors as nonverbal cues, motivation, and sociocultural roles. (p 44)

According to Bloom and Lahey (1978), the language system is described by three constituent parts: *form, content,* and *use.*

Language as a system

The form of language. Language form includes three of the parameters of language. Phonology is the sound system of language and includes the linguistic rules governing the various ways that sounds are able to be combined. In English, for example, we can combine the phonemes *s, e, e, r, t,* and *t* to form the word *street.* It is impossible, however, to form an acceptable word using the phonemes *k, w, k, y,* and *e.* In a similar manner, a linguistic rule system governs morphology or the formation of words as units. Morphemes, the least meaningful *units* of language, provide this structure. For example, the word *pig* contains *three* phonemes arranged in the configuration of a recognizable word. These three phonemes combine to form one morpheme (i.e., the word *pig*). The phoneme *s,* as an isolated unit, has no morphological or grammatical significance. When used in combination with the previous example, however, the meaning of *pig* (singular) is changed to that of *pigs* (plural). Here the phoneme *s* has changed into the morpheme *-s* which is a plural marker and provides additional grammatical meaning. Thus the plural word *pigs* contains two morphemes.

The third parameter of language commonly included in discussions of language form is syntax. Syntax is also governed by linguistic rules and is commonly described as the word order of grammatical sentences. The English language has very specific rules that dictate how a series of words may be combined to form a sentence. For example, the words *he, going, to, nap, a, take,* and *is* must be arranged in the specific order *He + is + going + to + take + a + nap* to have accurate syntactic (grammatical) meaning as a declarative sentence. On the other hand, the same series of words may form a yes/no question when arranged in the order *Is + he + going + to + take + a + nap.* The meaning of the two example sentences varies according to the two options available for the arrangement of the individual words into a grammatical series.

The underlying meaning of these sample sentences is only a part of syntax in that it pertains to the acceptable relationships among the constituent words. While this is usually obvious with short, concrete sentences, it is more difficult to separate word meaning from sentence meaning in complex or embedded sentences. The content of language is intricately related to the interpretation of many higher level grammatical structures. For example, the sentence *The boy, who is taking a nap, will go to the park with Joey and his mother when he wakes up* contains words that are easily understood by most school-age children. The length and complexity of the semantic/syntactic structure (content/form), however, may cause some children to misinterpret the meaning. These children might think that Joey or his mother are taking a nap and be utterly perplexed with the possibility that there is reference to three persons. Other children might be confused about *who* is going to the park and *when* they are going.

The content of language. Semantics is defined as the content of language, including both the meaning of individual words and the meaning of word combinations in sentences. Typically, we have tended to ignore the meaning of sentences or series of sentences and referred to semantics as the meaning of individual words. The dictionary meaning of isolated words is insufficient when considering our previous example word, *pig*. In a classroom a *pig* is identified as a farm animal, and usually some reference is made about a "cleanliness factor." However, it is not at all difficult for the reader to identify other "unteachable" meanings of this word!

Young children acquire word meanings in situationally specific contexts and then expand these meanings through repeated exposure to additional contexts. Older children continue to expand their semantic repertoires as they begin to understand jokes, metaphors, and ambiguities. The "here and now" environment of early language acquisition becomes increasingly context-free as school-age children are exposed to the semantic demands of the academic curriculum (Berlin, Blank, & Rose, 1980; Nelson, 1985; Simon, 1985; Wallach & Lee, 1980).

The functions of language. In order to conceptualize language as a complete system we must be able to see the "whole." The complete system includes the *form* of language (phonology, morphology, syntax), the *content* of language (semantics), and the *use* of language (pragmatics). Pragmatics is a sociolinguistic system in that language use is both situationally and culturally dependent. From the very earliest stages of language acquisition, the intentions of communication are important. Babies and toddlers concerned with concrete, immediate events frequently initiate communication by requesting desired objects or actions. Older children continue to develop sociolinguistic (pragmatic) skills. This is evidenced both in their interpersonal relationships and in their ability to decipher the language of the classroom. The historical emphasis on language structure as opposed to language use has previously limited our focus and thus our understanding of language as a system. Effective use of language for communication requires both a competency with language form and content and a knowledge of communicative variations in language use.

As Creaghead and Tattershall (1985, pp 108–109) have so aptly pointed out, children must have routines or scenarios for social interaction. These include communicative strategies for interacting with peers, teachers, and principals. As children progress through the elementary years, they not only refine rules for conversation, but also learn appropriate structures for more formal group discussion and debate. Both conversation and classroom interaction demand that students maintain organization, coherence, and continuity.

Summary of the Definition of Language

The following list summarizes the definition of language:

1. Language is a dynamic system, including content, form, and use.
2. Language is culturally dependent.
3. Language is developmental.
4. Normal language development involves the interdependence of biological, social, cognitive, and environmental factors.
5. Each parameter of language is rule-governed.
6. The parameters of language (phonology, morphology, syntax, semantics, and pragmatics) have not been ranked in terms of importance. An effective, efficient oral communication system requires mastery of all the parameters.

QUESTIONS FOR DISCUSSION

1. What groups of students are identified as "high-incidence" language-deficient students? Which of these groups are at-risk for academic/social failure?
2. What is language?
3. What are language deficiencies (disorders)?
4. What are four examples of deficient language?
5. What is the classroom teacher's role in the IEPC process?
6. What is the meaning of "mutual intelligibility"?
7. How do language deficiencies affect classroom behaviors?
8. What is the "language of schooling"?
9. What are three intervention techniques that will be useful in your classroom?
10. Explain the relationship between language for academics and language for socialization.

REFERENCES

American Speech–Language–Hearing Association (1982). Definition of language disorders. *ASHA, 24*, 949–950

American Speech–Language–Hearing Association (1982). Position statement on language learning disabilities. *ASHA, 24*, 937–944

American Speech–Language–Hearing Association (1983). Definition of language. *ASHA, 25*, 44

Aram DM, Ekelman BL, & Nation JE (1984). Preschoolers with language disorders: 10 years later. *Journal of Speech and Hearing Research, 27*, 232–244

Baker L, & Cantwell DP (1982). Developmental, social and behavioral characteristics of speech and language disordered children. *Child Psychiatry and Human Development, 12,* 195–206

Baker L, Cantwell DP, & Mattison RE (1980). Behavior problems in children with pure speech disorders and children with combined speech and language disorders. *Journal of Abnormal Child Psychology, 8,* 245–256

Berlin LJ, Blank M, & Rose SA (1980). The language of instruction: The hidden complexities. *Topics in Language Disorders, 1* (1), 47–58

Bernstein, B (1971). *Class, codes and control I: Theoretical studies towards a sociology of language.* London: Routeledge & Kegan Paul

Bloom RM (1980). The role of language therapy in school based intervention programs for behaviorally disordered latency age children. *Dissertations Abstracts, 41* (4), 1528A–1529A, Order No. DDJ80-22808

Bloom L, & Lahey M (1978). *Language development and language disorders.* New York: John Wiley & Sons

Blue CM (1975). The marginal communicator. *Language, Speech and Hearing Services in Schools, 6,* 32–38

Boyce NL, & Lord-Larson V (1983). *Adolescents' communication: Development and disorders.* Eau Claire, WI: Thinking Ink Publications

Butler KG (1984). The language of the schools. *ASHA, 34,* 31–35

Cazden C (1973). Problems for education: Language as curriculum, context, and learning environment. *American Academy of Arts and Sciences, 102,* 135–148

Creaghead NA, & Tattershall SS (1985). Observation and assessment of classroom pragmatic skills. In CS Simon (Ed.), *Communication skills and classroom success: Assessment of language-learning disabled students.* San Diego: College-Hill Press 105–131

Damico J, & Oller Jr JW (1980). Pragmatic versus morphological/syntactic criteria for language referrals. *Language, Speech and Hearing Services in Schools, 11,* 85–94

Danziger RK (1971). *Socialization.* Harmondsworth, England: Penguin Books

Fujiki M, & Brinton B (1984). Supplementing language therapy: Working with the classroom teacher. *Language, Speech and Hearing Services in Schools, 15,* 98–109

Garrard KR (1979). The changing role of speech and hearing professionals in public education. *ASHA, 21* (2), 91–98

Greenacre P (1950). General problems of acting out. *Psychoanalytic Quarterly, 19,* 455–467

Gualteri CT, Koriath U, Van Bourgondien M, & Saleeby U (1983). Language disorders in children referred for psychiatric services. *Journal of the American Academy of Child Psychiatry, 22* (2), 165–171

Hymes D (1972). Introduction. In C Cazden, D John & D Hymes (Eds.), *Functions of language in the classroom.* New York: Teachers College Press, Columbia University, xi–lvii

Johnson DJ, & Myklebust HR (1967). *Learning disabilities: Educational Principles and practices.* Orlando, FL: Grune & Stratton

Kagan J, & Tulkin SR (1971). Social class differences in childrearing during the first year. In R Schaffer (Ed.), *The origins of human social relations.* Orlando, FL: Academic Press, 165–186

Lerner JA, Inui TS, Trupin EW, & Douglas E (1985). Preschool behavior can predict future psychiatric disorders. *Journal of the American Academy of Child Psychiatry, 24,* 42–48

Mattison RE, Cantwell DP, & Baker L (1980). Dimensions of behavior in children with speech and language disorders. *Journal of Abnormal Child Psychology, 8,* 323–338

Menyuk P (1983). Language development and reading. In TM Gallagher & CA Prutting (Eds.), *Pragmatic assessment and intervention issues in language.* San Diego: College-Hill Press, 151–170

Naremore RC, & Hipskind NM (1979). Responses to the language of educable mentally retarded and normal children: Stereotypes and judgments. *Language, Speech and Hearing Services in Schools, 10,* 27–34

Nelson NW (1985). Teacher talk and child listening—fostering a better match. In CS Simon (Ed.), *Communication skills and classroom success: Assessment of language learning disabled students.* San Diego: College-Hill Press, 65–102

Olson DR (1980). The language of schooling. *Topics in Language Disorders, 2* (4), 1–12

Prutting CA (1979). Process: The action of moving forward progressively from one point to another on the way to completion. *Journal of Speech and Hearing Disorders, 44,* 3–20

Randall D, Reynell J, & Curwen M (1974). A study of language development in a sample of three year old children. *British Journal of Disorders of Communication, 9,* 3–16

Rexford EU (1966). A developmental approach to problems of acting out: A symposium. *Monographs of the Journal of the American Academy of Child Psychiatry,* Vol. 1. New York: International Universities Press

Schaffer R (1977). *Mothering.* Cambridge, MA: Harvard University Press

Simon CS (1985). The language-learning disabled student: Description and assessment implications. In CS Simon (Ed.), *Communication skills and classroom success: Assessment of language-learning disabled students.* San Diego: College-Hill Press, 1–40, 53

Stevenson J, Richman N, & Graham R (1985). Behavior problems and language abilities at three years and behavioral deviance at eight years. *Journal of Child Psychology and Psychiatry, 26* (2), 215–230

Wallach GP, & Lee AP (1980). So you want to know what to do with language disabled children above the age of six. *Topics in Language Disorders, 1* (1), 99–113

Wiig EH (1984). Language disabilities in adolescents: A question of cognitive strategies. *Topics in Language Disorders, 4* (2), 41–58

9

Language Differences

Nicholas G. Bountress

EDITOR'S INTRODUCTION

In this chapter, Dr. Bountress discusses the varied problems inherent in the classroom in which there are different dialect speakers. While it should be recognized that these same problems occur to speakers of other dialects, the author describes children who speak in black English.

Teaching strategies with respect to these children have been generally ineffective. What should the teacher do? How should the teacher react to these nonstandard speakers? These themes are addressed by Dr. Bountress.

Nicholas Bountress is a prolific writer and researcher and is well-respected by his peers. His research on social dialects has focused on the professional, educational, and clinical implications of language differences.

EDUCATIONAL FAILURE AND CULTURAL DISADVANTAGE

While issues regarding the education of minority children, in particular black children, have been of major concern throughout the history of the United States, it was not until the 1950s that significant numbers of American educators suggested that the fault for the educational failure of such children might lie within the educational system and not with the children. For decades, the nation's schools had demonstrated a tendency for racially-based tracking, the process by which educationally disadvantaged or culturally disadvantaged children found themselves in academic groupings that suggested that they had a lowered capacity for learning. Such groupings led to decreased teacher expectations for such children, which led to increased academic failure and increased minority dropout rates from public schools. The educational research that frequently described these occurrences laid the blame not with the system but with genetic and environmental factors that supposedly

ORAL COMMUNICATION PROBLEMS
IN CHILDREN AND ADOLESCENTS
Copyright © 1988 by Grune & Stratton, Inc.

ISBN 0-8089-1887-7

operated within disadvantaged populations. If minority students were failing in schools because of lack of environmental stimulation and/or genetic inferiority, it followed that the schools could do little to raise such children's level of academic achievement. During the 1950s, concerned educators suggested that intelligence tests and tests of academic achievement failed to take into account the intrinsic cultural biases of these measures and failed to consider the effect of cultural influences upon each child. These educators suggested the need for investigating the nature of intelligence tests, individualizing instruction, and establishing educational objectives in terms of the abilities and needs of students. Furthermore, many educators emphasized the role that public schools must play in introducing teachers and students to the variety of ethnic and cultural lifestyles, developing higher expectations for minority students, and helping minority students to develop positive attitudes toward their own cultures. In addition, it was recommended that teachers become aware of the racist assumptions that underlie much social research and develop greater sensitivity toward ethnic cultures.

The implications of these changes in attitudes among educators during the 1950s were of no small significance, particularly as they related to the world outside of the classroom. Williams (1970) suggested that such changes in perspective are of significance in disrupting the "poverty cycle." This cycle is characterized by developmental disadvantage, which is frequently associated with being raised in families that suffer from economic disadvantage. This, in turn, leads to educational disadvantage, or failure in the classroom, which leads to employment disadvantage, or the inability to qualify only for jobs with limited economic and professional benefits. The cycle is completed when employment disadvantage leads to further economic and developmental disadvantages. As Williams has suggested, the location in the cycle that is most susceptible to intervention is educational disadvantage. It is at this point that educators can exert their influence to break the cycle, first by identifying those variables that lead to failure and then by taking appropriate action.

Educational Disadvantage and Language Usage

Among the variables that have been described as contributing to educational disadvantage is language, which has probably been the issue that has been least understood and most intensely debated. Arguments concerning the influence of linguistic variables on the educational failure of children, particularly black children, from the lower socioeconomic level have placed educators, researchers, and other professionals into two opposing positions. One position espouses the point of view that the language of lower socioeconomic-level children is deficient, resulting from genetic inferiority and/or cultural deprivation. The second position, which was developed during the early 1960s, argued that the language of such children is different from standard English, but is a logical, rule-governed and structurally complex linguistic system. These two points of view have come to be regarded as the *language deficit* and *language difference* positions.

Language Deficit Position

The language deficit position was an attempt to describe the linguistic abilities of all lower socioeconomic-level children, but has been used most frequently to describe the language of black children from the lower socioeconomic level. Prior to the 1960s, the deficit position was the most commonly accepted position of educators, and it continues to be accepted by many professionals. The basic tenets of this position are that the linguistic variations of lower socioeconomic-level children are ungrammatical, illogical, communicatively limited, and poor approximations of standard English, and that these variations are products of linguistic impoverishment due to genetic differences and environmental-cultural factors. The research studies that formed the basis for the deficit position focused upon four major linguistic parameters: vocabulary, speech–sound development, mean length of response, and speech–sound discrimination. These studies were structured so that black and/or lower socioeconomic-level children and white and/or middle socioeconomic-level children were compared on one parameter through the administration of a test to both sets of children. The results were then compared to ascertain which group performed better.

Language Difference Position

While the preceding research gave considerable support to the perspectives of many educators and researchers, there was a marked increase in the criticism of such studies by researchers who were sensitive to major research design flaws that were common to deficit position studies. Foremost among these criticisms, and seemingly most obvious, was the fact that many of the evaluative procedures or tools that were utilized contained linguistically-biased items. Based upon normative data gained from white, middle-class populations, such tools did not allow for any linguistic variations that consistently conformed to grammatical and phonologic rules of nonstandard dialects. As has been noted by numerous researchers, when such variables are removed, there are no significant language differences between blacks and whites. Another major problem with these studies was that little information was gained directly, the researchers relying upon questionnaires and other less reliable means of collecting data. Furthermore, vocabulary sampling and measurements of mean length of response are procedures insufficiently expansive to allow inferences regarding linguistic mastery and potential. With these concerns in mind, sociolinguistic researchers in the 1960s undertook a number of studies in the major urban centers of the United States that radically departed from the purpose of previous studies. Shunning the prior tendency for black-white comparative studies, these researchers focused on descriptions of the syntactic and phonologic variations of black children without comparison to the language of white middle-class children and without reliance upon evaluative tools or procedures that could be considered to be linguistically biased. This approach allowed for the investigation of black children's language with regard to their own linguistic communities, thereby allowing for more realistic and utilitarian descriptions of linguistic normalcy and deviation. By varying their perspective in this manner, these researchers often described as language differences those characteristics of syntax and phonology that earlier writers had described as deficient.

The above mentioned urban language studies were conducted in New York City, Washington, D.C., Chicago, and Detroit, among others, and provided evidence that indicated the presence of a corpus of rule-governed linguistic characteristics that was consistent among black English speakers regardless of geographic area. While black English speakers in a particular area were not found to produce all the characteristics described in the above studies, and, in fact, used regional variations that were, in some cases, characteristic of other American dialects, the characteristics described are found in varying degrees in the speech and language of most blacks from the lower socioeconomic level. The information gained from the urban language studies has had a significant and far-reaching influence on the attitudes of many professionals and has served as the basis for legal decisions, such as the Ann Arbor decision of 1979, which will be discussed later, and the attitudes of professionals as expressed in the position papers of organizations such as the Linguistic Society of America (LSA, 1972) and the American Speech–Language–Hearing Association (ASHA, 1983). The LSA's position paper represented the consensus of modern linguists and presented their opinion that no one language or dialect can be regarded as being significantly more complex than another in its grammatical structure. Furthermore, the LSA indicated that linguists have not discovered a speech community with a native language that can be described as deficient, and that nonstandard dialects are fully formed languages with all the grammatical structure necessary for logical thought. The position paper of ASHA, the professional organization that establishes the minimal standards for the training of professionals in the field of speech, language, and hearing disorders, reflected the position of the LSA. Of practical significance, the ASHA position stated that speech–language clinicians must be able to recognize dialectal linguistic features, differentiate such features from pathologic variations, and have a clear understanding that dialectal variations are grammatically and phonologically correct for the child's environment and, thereby, not in need of correction. These perspectives, developed and espoused by professionals whose principal purpose has been to study the normal and aberrant development of language, are of significance for the classroom teacher whose influence upon linguistically different children may be the single most critical factor in their educational success as well as in the fulfillment of their individual potential.

THE CLASSROOM TEACHER AND THE LANGUAGE-DIFFERENT CHILD

Classroom Failure and Language Differences

The frequent academic failure and disproportionate school drop-out rates of lower socioeconomic-level children and, in particular, lower socioeconomic-level black children, indicate that the nation's schools have fallen short in their mission to maximize the potential of and intellectually stimulate and guide students from all cultural and economic backgrounds. Numerous reasons have been suggested for the above phenomena, with one of the more compelling being the negative communicative environment in which the language-different child interacts in the classroom setting. The dynamics of this interaction have been a source of conjecture and debate for many years. Some researchers, such as Cohn (1959), Caplan and Ruble (1964), and Blank and Solomon (1969), have suggested that the initial barrier that minority, particularly black, children must face in the schools is having to adjust to the fact that classroom activities are transacted in standard English. It was theorized that linguistic interference created by differences between the home and school dialects resulted in comprehension problems for children, often causing them to misinterpret information presented by the classroom teacher. However, later researchers such as Frentz (1971) and Ramsey (1972) concluded that black children had little or no difficulty in code switching between dialects. It was also widely believed that, as has been noted in the arguments of the "language deficit" theorists, black children's substandard linguistic abilities were a product of inferior intellectual capacity. However, the results of the urban language studies as reflected in the position of the LSA position paper of 1972 forcefully advanced the arguments that the minimal ability to speak and learn any human language requires a high order of intelligence and that conclusions regarding intelligence based upon the results of traditional standardized tests are, for the most part, groundless. If, then, lower socioeconomic-level black children were not to be regarded as being deficient in intelligence and linguistic abilities, then the factor or factors that led to ongoing classroom failure still needed to be identified. It has become increasingly evident that these factors are related to the conflict between the child's culture and the standards and values of the predominantly middle-class school. Loban (1968), for example, has noted that language and social caste are inextricably interwoven and that the language-different child's oral communication reflects that lower status. Therefore, children whose awareness of their lower-class status are accentuated by their awareness of their language difference may be reticent to participate in classroom discussions even if they have no difficulty in comprehending and using standard English. Such children must also deal with the dilemma of selecting which mode of verbal response to use. Do they use dialectal responses and risk criticism by teachers and middle-class peers or use standard English and risk the ridicule of their friends? A third option is remaining mute to avoid any disparagement. Given the large number of studies that describe the lack of verbosity of lower-class black children, it would appear that such an option is a common choice. However, children who are able to overcome their reticence to speak in class must also overcome the barriers posed by teacher attitudes. Cohn (1959) stated that class antagonism on the part of teachers is one of the most powerful factors contributing to the feelings of alienation that lower-class children experience in school settings. That antagonism may be consciously or unconsciously transmitted by the teacher's verbal and nonverbal responses to the child's language. If the unwary or insensitive teacher ridicules or harshly corrects the child, it may discourage attempts at further communication and damage the child's self-concept. Furthermore, if the teacher perceives the child's dialect as being deficient and, therefore, indicative of lowered intelligence, that fact may be communicated to the child who fulfills the teacher's expectations of failure. It is not uncommon for children to respond to such attitudes by performing below their capabilities and, eventually, losing interest in formal schooling. Early intervention is necessary to stem the possibility of failure or the tendency to drop out of school, and must be implemented by school administrators and specialists as well as classroom teachers. Foremost in this intervention process is the necessity for becoming sensitive to the cultural and linguistic background of each child and creating an atmosphere in which the child feels free to express himself or herself without the threat of overt or covert penalty. From an oral communication perspective, these goals can be attained when professionals understand that nonstandard dialects are complex and rule-governed and as indicative of intellectual capacity as is standard English.

The Ann Arbor Decision

While it may be that such changes in attitude may spontaneously occur in classroom teachers and others, it is, unfortunately, more likely that such attitudes will only be changed when legal action is taken by concerned individuals and policy changes are legally mandated. While a number of legal decisions have been successful in clarifying the problem of language differences in the schools, none has had the national impact of a federal suit filed in Michigan's Eastern District Court in 1979. This landmark ruling, *Martin Luther King Elementary School Children, et al., Plaintiffs, v. Ann Arbor School District, Defendant*, has come to be regarded as the "Ann Arbor Decision" and has established a precedent for the recognition of nonstandard English as well as for the delineation of responsibilities of local school districts. The decision was the result of a suit initiated by black parents and their attorneys who claimed that the children's use of dialect interfered with their equal participation in academic programs. Specifically, the attorneys for the plaintiffs claimed that the school had failed to recognize the pervasive use of dialect and failed to understand its influence upon the teaching of reading and learning of standard English. Furthermore, the plaintiffs argued that the school's failure to respond appropriately resulted in the black student's lack of normal academic progress and inappropriate grade placement. Substantiation of the parents' argument was provided by a team of experts comprised of linguists and educators who discussed the current state of knowledge regarding nonstandard English, the rule-governed features of black English, and the effect of negative teacher attitudes on the language-different speaker.

The presiding judge in the Ann Arbor decision concluded that, while the teachers at King School may not have been overtly critical of the children's dialect, they did not take it into account when teaching standard English. In the opinion of the court, failing to consider the influence of the native dialect created a barrier to the learning of standard English that ultimately led to difficulties in learning to read. The decision rendered by the court required the defendant to submit a plan that would help the King School teachers to identify black English features and to use that information to develop a program for teaching students to read standard English. The plan submitted by the Ann Arbor Board of Education included a Formal Instructional Component, and a Classroom Application Component, as well as a new reading program. The Formal Instructional Component included 20 hours of formal instruction for the teachers by a team of language art consultants, while the Classroom Application Component incorporated the use of the instructional content in classroom settings. The objectives of the instructional component were as follows:

1. recognize generally the basic features of a language system as they apply to dialect differences
2. be able to describe in general the concept of a dialect and dialect differences within the English language
3. be sensitive to the value judgments about dialect differences that people often make and communicate to others
4. be able to describe the basic linguistic features of black English as it contrasts with standard English
5. show appreciation for the history and background of black English
6. recognize readily children and adults speaking the black English dialect
7. be able to identify, without prompting, the specific linguistic features by which they recognized a speaker of black English dialect
8. be able to discuss knowledgeably the important linguistic issues in code-switching between black English and standard written English
9. be able to identify possible instructional strategies that can be used to aid children in code-switching between black English and standard English
10. use miscue analysis strategies to distinguish between a dialect shift and a decoding mistake when analyzing an oral reading sample
11. be able to describe a variety of language experience activities that can be used to complement the linguistic basal reader program

The objectives for the instructional component developed for teachers at King School should also serve as frames of reference for any classroom teacher, as well as any other professional, who is responsible for facilitating the educational progress of language-different children. First, and perhaps foremost, these objectives underscore the need for understanding the basic tenets of the previously discussed language-deficit–language-different argument and the research that supported both arguments. Secondly, the objectives underscore the need for the classroom teacher to develop an understanding of the grammatical and phonologic features that characterize the language of children in their particular school. Descriptions of these features, such as those discussed earlier in this chapter, provide reliable evidence of the structural validity of dialects and provide a basis for instilling a sensitivity toward and acceptance of spoken language patterns that may be foreign to the ear of middle-class speakers. Such knowledge also improves the likelihood of better communication between teacher and student and alerts the teacher to linguistic barriers that may be present in classroom activities and materials. With regard to the latter concern, the available research should alert the teacher to the linguistic biases of most traditional tests of intelligence and academic achievement, whose distorted conclusions may result in the inaccurate and destructive labeling of language-different children as slow learners, language-disordered, learning disabled, or worse. Knowledge of the child's language can, in conjunction with information provided by the school speech–language clinician, aid the teacher in designing programs that stimulate verbalization and insure the development of speaking and writing skills (Baskervill, 1977). In short, such information, when understood and applied to learning situations by the classroom teacher, can enhance the opportunity for academic adjustment and success by language-different children.

TEACHING STANDARD ENGLISH TO THE LANGUAGE-DIFFERENT CHILD

Responsibilities of the Classroom Teacher

When the classroom teacher has studied the available research regarding the language-different–language-deficit argument, gained an understanding of the grammatical and phonologic characteristics of the child's language, developed an appreciation of the complexity and validity of the child's language, and developed a sensitivity toward the child's cultural heritage, the intervention process can be initiated. It is in the best interests of the teacher and language-different child if this process is the product of collaboration between the teacher and speech-language clinician as well as other professionals who possess an understanding of language differences. Typically, speech–language clinicians are best suited for developing such programs because of their training in differentiating language differences from language disorders, developing programs based upon sound theoretic foundations, and implementing such programs with a wide variety of children. This kind of expertise is critical, not only because intervention programs must be methodically structured and implemented, but because the target behaviors must be clearly delineated. In the case of the language-different child, target behaviors are understood to be dialectal features and not speech and language disorders. Because speech–language clinicians are specifically trained to make this differentiation between language differences and true disorders, their expertise is invaluable in program planning.

Alternative Approaches in Language Intervention with Language-Different Children

There is no unanimity regarding the philosophy or design of intervention as applied to the teaching of standard English to language-different children. For example, Wolfram and Fasold (1974) cite three potential alternatives related to the intervention process: eradication of the dialect and teaching of standard English, training in bidialectalism, and retention of the nonstandard dialect without the teaching of standard English. Bidialectalism involves the teaching of standard English while advocating a respect for the native dialect, and appears to be the most logical, humane, and appropriate approach. Eradicationism has been practiced by classroom teachers and other educational personnel who have not recognized dialectal characteristics, nor understood the language difference argument, nor had sufficient knowledge of even the most rudimentary aspects of linguistic theory. The argument against the eradication viewpoint is that, apart from the damaging effect that such an approach has upon the child's self-concept, it is illogical in the sense that, if dialects are different and not deficient, professionals cannot correct something that is already correct. The third alternative, retention of the native dialect, is highly controversial. It recommends that the dialect not be changed but that the negative attitudes of persons be altered. Based upon the wholly acceptable premise that dialects are not deficient, this theory, nevertheless, makes the inaccurate assumption that it is easier to alter people's negative attitudes than it is to teach a child to become bidialectal. Given the persuasive literature that describes the barriers posed by insensitive teachers and employers, the academic and economic futures of many language-different children could be sacrificed while waiting for a more perfect world to evolve.

Bidialectalism

While bidialectalism is the approach espoused by most practitioners in the fields of sociolinguistics and speech–language pathology, it should be observed that even advocates of this approach are not entirely in agreement regarding when it is appropriate to initiate such programs. Some professionals believe that dialect speakers should be taught standard English when they are sufficiently aware of the need for it, or approximately the late junior high school years. Advocates of early intervention argue that the purpose of developing bidialectal programs is to provide children with a less stigmatized tool for verbal expression that can be used to facilitate success in the classroom. To wait until the middle teenage years to implement bidialectal programs would negate this purpose and would ignore the fact that the early school years represent a period in which children are remarkably facile in their ability to acquire a wide variety of language behaviors. Furthermore, the results of early intervention programs developed and applied by Adler (1979), Feigenbaum (1970), Johnson (1971) and others indicate that bidialectalism can be effectively taught as early as the kindergarten years and results in increments in both the quality and quantity of verbal expression and in classroom participatory behaviors.

As mentioned in the previous section, bidialectalism involves the teaching of standard English while advocating a respect for the native dialect. The format that is typically utilized is based upon foreign-language pedagogy and incorporates the use of contrastive analysis. Specifically, this approach compares standard English phonologic and grammatical features with those of the child's dialect and is structured so that children may see how their linguistic features differ from those of standard English. The goal of this method is to teach standard English through a graduated series of exercises that incorporate contrastive techniques. While the exercises included in this section appear to be quite simple in structure and easily applicable to a classroom setting, the selection of grammatical and phonologic features and the manner in which they are integrated into specific exercises require a fundamental understanding of the child's language and procedures for sequencing concepts and basic learning theory. The following examples are based upon procedures described by Feigenbaum (1970) and are representative and not exhaustive samplings of contrastive exercises. While they utilize black English features, the basic procedures can be utilized with a variety of language-different populations.

Preparatory Phase

The initial phase of intervention requires a careful assessment of the grammatical and phonologic features of the child's speech and language for the purpose of identifying targets for contrastive analysis. This analysis is best conducted by a speech–language clinician or other professional with a strong background in the areas of language variation and development. Sampling of the child's language should focus on the use of formal tests of grammar and phonology, as well as the elicitation of imitated and informal spontaneous utterances.

This phase should also include discussions of dialects and, specifically, as Feigenbaum (1970) notes, that dialects are different not deficient. Exercises should focus on analyzing the regional characteristics that are apparent in the language of television broadcasters, actors in selected roles, and characters in books. Discussions should also focus on the appropriateness of a specified language or dialect in certain situations, for example that there is a "school" language and a "home/street" language. At all times, this phase should have as its purpose the nurturing of respect for language differences.

Word Discrimination

The following is an example of a word discrimination drill using standard English (SE) and black English (BE) rules:

Teacher Stimulus	*Child Response*
1. Masks (SE)—Masses (BE)	different
2. Masses (BE)—Masses (BE)	same
3. Masks (SE)—Masks (SE)	same

In this drill, the teacher presents stimuli that are combinations of standard and nonstandard English and the children must indicate their ability to differentiate them by saying "same" or "different." The word "masses" is a common dialectal production of "masks."

Sentence Discrimination

The following is an example of a sentence discrimination drill:

Teacher Stimulus	*Child Response*
1. They wear masses (BE)— They wear masks (SE).	different
2. They wear masks (SE)— They wear masks (SE).	same

In this drill, the teacher presents stimuli that are similar to those in the word drill except that key words are placed in sentences, and the child responds with "same" or "different."

Home—School Discrimination

The following is an example of a drill in which the child must identify whether the stimuli are representative of home (dialectal) or school (standard English) language:

Teacher Stimulus	*Child Response*
1. They wear masses (BE).	home
2. John play hard (BE).	home
3. John plays hard (SE).	school

Translation Drills

The following is an example of a translation drill:

Teacher Stimulus	*Child Response*
1. He drinks soup (SE).	He drink soup (BE).
2. He plays baseball (SE).	He play baseball (BE).
3. She drives a Buick (SE).	She drive a Buick (BE).
4. She drive a Buick (BE).	She drives a Buick (SE).
5. He drink soup (BE).	He drinks soup (SE).

This drill requires the child to not only translate a standard English stimulus into nonstandard but also the nonstandard into standard. Focusing on only one feature at a time, in this case the third person singular verb form, the child is provided with opportunities to listen to and produce standard English stimuli as well as nonstandard stimuli. The exercises can be varied systematically and in a variety of ways. For example, the singular pronoun (he, she) form can be replaced by a plural (they) stimulus or another entirely different target feature. An example of the latter would be the following translation drill in which plural forms appear:

Teacher Stimulus	*Child Response*
1. John has three car (BE).	John has three cars (SE).
2. John has three cars (SE).	John has three car (BE).

Response Drills

Response drills provide the child with the opportunity to use the contrastive methodology in a more natural context. An example of a response drill is the following, in which the child must negate the teacher's stimulus with a dialectally consistent response:

Teacher Stimulus	*Child Response*
1. John play baseball (BE).	No, he don't (BE).
2. The teacher read the story (BE).	No, she don't (BE).
3. John plays baseball (SE).	No, he doesn't (SE).

The response drills provide a framework for developing a variety of exercises that can be greatly varied in complexity. For example, the teacher can present a stimulus using dialectal or standard English forms and require the child to use a broad range of responses from affirmation ("Yes, he does." / "Yes, he do.") and interrogation ("Does he?" / "Do he?") to changes in verb tense, plurality, and many others.

The drills described by Feigenbaum and others have been developed to teach standard English by building on the child's own linguistic repertoire. Such an approach not only can provide the children with an opportunity to observe their own linguistic features, but also can engender an appreciation of the consistency of those features. When employed by the sensitive and knowledgeable teacher, these activities can do much to provide the language-different child with a tool for survival and success in the middle-class school setting.

APPENDIX

Grammatical and Phonologic Features of Black English

The major urban language studies conducted in the 1960s in New York City, Detroit, Chicago, Washington, D.C., and elsewhere by researchers such as Stewart (1964), Wolfram (1969), McDavid (1970), Fasold and Wolfram (1972), and Labov (1975), among others, spawned a multitude of related studies that examined the origins of black English, the linguistic biases of intelligence, achievement, speech and language tests, the communicative environment of the middle-class school, and the role of educators in helping or hindering lower socioeconomic-level children's adjustment to educational settings. These studies also established more reliable procedures for studying the linguistic variations of speakers of nonstandard dialects. Specifically, in-depth descriptions of the language of linguistically different children were obtained through personal interviews and language sampling in the subjects' environment conducted by interviewers with sensitivity toward and an understanding of the subjects' culture and linguistic variations. While the grammatical and phonologic data that have been gathered through such procedures have been invaluable to the sociolinguist and speech–language pathologist, dissemination to the classroom teacher is of critical importance. It is the classroom teacher who has the most significant influence on students on an ongoing basis and, therefore, is the professional who must have not only a tolerance for language differences, but an understanding of the rules and characteristics that differentiate dialects such as black English from standard English. Such understanding is critical if the classroom teacher is to communicate effectively with nonwhite and/or non-middle-class children and promote their positive adjustment to the classroom environment. The following discussion focuses on the grammatical and phonologic features of black English as derived from the above mentioned urban language studies.

Grammatical Features

Past forms. Descriptions of black English have noted the omission of both /t/ and /d/ in final positions of words in which the *-ed* suffix was used to denote the past tense or past participle. As is also noted in numerous studies, however, the omissions are often due to pronunciation characteristics that are found in the dialect. For example, for situations in which the addition of *-ed* results in a cluster of either voiced (*moved, robbed*) or unvoiced (*wrapped, kicked*) consonants, the final /t/ or /d/ that signifies the *-ed* suffix may be removed. Such an occurrence may produce a sentence such as, *He rob the bank last week.*

Perfective constructions. Researchers have described changes that occur in black English with respect to perfective constructions, particularly in the present perfect and completive aspects. A common occurrence in the use of present perfect constructions is the omission of forms of *have* as an auxiliary in the contracted form, giving sentences such as, *I seen the car.* Black English also has a completive aspect that is formed by the use of *done* plus a past form, which allows for the production of such sentences as *I done tried.*

Third person singular present tense. One of the more common characteristics of the language of black children from economically disadvantaged areas occurs in the production of the third person singular present tense, particularly in regard to the *-s* and *-es* suffixes. Researchers have noted that the *-s* and *-es* suffixes are frequently absent, but emphasize that this is not a careless omission and that those suffixes are simply not part of the dialectal grammar. Such omissions, therefore, may allow for the production of such sentences as, *He walk* and *The man talk.* Hypercorrection may cause the speaker to use the *-s* suffix with the first person (*I walks*) and second person (*You walks*) singular and plural, and third person plural (*They walks*).

Fasold and Wolfram have also noted that the omission of the *-s* suffix may result in the substitution of *have* for *has.* They note that the verb *have* is unique because the combination of *have* and *-s* results in *has* rather than *haves,* and since the *-s* suffix does not exist in the dialect, the verb remains *have.* Such an occurrence is described as the reason for the production of sentences such as, *He have a bike.*

Invariant "be."   In black English, *be* assumes a relatively fixed position and occurs as a main verb in a variety of contexts. Therefore, such sentences as *He be going* and *They be going* may occur. The word *be* may also be used to indicate habitual activity, for example, *He be working* (in his job at the Post Office) while deletion may indicate momentary activity, as in *He working* (right now).

Absence of forms of "to be."   Absence of forms of *to be* are common among black children and adults, and is referred to as *zero copula*. While *are* is rarely produced in black English, *is* may be omitted in any situation in which the contracted form occurs in standard English, as in *He going home.*

Plural and possessive suffixes.   Both plural and possessive suffixes frequently are omitted in the language of black speakers from the lower socioeconomic level. As Fasold and Wolfram and others have stated, that instead of the *'s* suffix to indicate possession, the mere positioning of words in the sentence is sufficient to indicate that one is the possessor and the other is the possessed, as in *John old man house.* Hypercorrection may account for confusion in the attachment of the *'s* suffix to proper names, as in *Bill's Wilson Store.*

A number of studies have also indicated that the plural *-s* suffix may also be absent in the language of black English speakers, resulting in sentences such as *Five car are outside.* The absence of the plural suffix, however, generally occurs more often in the language of the southern urban black than in the northern black.

Future constructions.   The use of *gonna* as a future indicator in black English very frequently occurs with deletion of forms of *to be*, giving *They gonna get you.* Furthermore, as a number of researchers have indicated, when the subject of the sentence is *I, gonna* can be reduced to *ngna*, as in *I ngna listen to you.* When *I* is not present as the subject of the sentence, the black English speaker may reduce *gonna* to *gon*, giving *They gon get you.*

Negative forms.   Black English speakers as well as speakers of other nonstandard American dialects frequently use *ain't* as a substitution for negative forms of the verb *to be* and forms of *have*. It should be noted that the listener may confuse the production of *ain't* with dialectal reductions of *don't* (*'on't*) and *didn't* (*'in't*), because of the small degree of phonologic distinctions between each of them that occurs in conversational speech. It should be understood, then, that seeming inconsistencies in the dialect speaker's use of *ain't* may be due more to phonologic assimilation than syntactic or semantic confusion.

In addition to *ain't* black English speakers frequently use multiple negation, for example, *I don't know nothing about it.* Therefore, while standard English does not allow for such constructions, black English allows negatives to be expressed more than once in a sentence. An in-depth analysis of placement rules for negatives is provided by Fasold and Shuy.

Pronominal apposition. While there is considerable variability in the use of pronouns in black English, one of the most common constructions is pronominal apposition. Used in many nonstandard dialects, pronominal apposition is characterized by the lack of deletion of the noun or noun phrase for which a pronoun is commonly substituted, giving *My brother, he bought a car* and *The Smiths, they're bad.*

Phonologic Features

"Th" sounds. One of the most commonly identified characteristics of black English is related to the change in the form of both voiced and voiceless *th* sounds. It should be emphasized again, as is the case with many black English features, that these changes in the form of *th* are common to other nonstandard dialects as well. Furthermore, the changes in the form of *th* are also regarded as characteristic of normal stages of phonologic development in standard English.

The most consistent changes in the form of *th* are substitution of /t/ for voiceless *th* and /d/ for voiced *th*. There is some variability, however, in such substitutions as a function of placement in a word. In initial position in words, these changes are likely to be common, giving *dem* and *doze* for *them* and *those* as well as *tanks* and *tinks* for *thanks* and *thinks*. One variation of this tendency occurs in initial *thr* words when /f/ is a frequent substitution, giving *froat* and *fred* for *throat* and *thread*.

In the medial position of words, the variability of choices for phoneme substitution increases. While /d/ and /t/ may be substituted for their voiced and unvoiced counterparts, the more frequently occurring variations are likely to be /f/ for unvoiced *th,* giving *nuffing* for *nothing,* and /v/ for voiced *th,* giving *lever* for *leather.* When a nasalized consonant phoneme follows the *th* sound, however, /t/ is often substituted, giving *matumatics* and *aritmutic* for *mathematics* and *arithmetic.*

In the final position of *th* words, /f/ and /v/ are the most frequent substitutions, giving *mouf* and *bref* for *mouth* and *breath,* and *breev* for *breathe.* Some of the same variability that occurs in standard English also occurs in black English, as is the case with the word *with* that may be produced with a voiced or voiceless *th* in final position in standard English, and as *wiv* or *wif* in black English.

Consonant clusters. Phonologic reduction of consonant clusters that occurs in the final position of words is a common occurrence in the language of black English speakers. Reduction is the process by which a phoneme is omitted from a word in compliance with specific linguistic rules. It should, therefore, be noted that such omissions are neither inconsistent nor haphazard. In black English, such reductions can only occur when both phonemes in the word-final consonant cluster are either voiced or voiceless. For example, in the words *chest* and *mask,* both cluster phonemes (*st* and *sk*) are voiceless; therefore, both words can be reduced, giving *ches'* and *mas'*. In the cases of *build* and *find,* both cluster phonemes (*ld* and *nd*) are voiced; therefore, both words can be reduced, giving *buil'* and *fin'*. It is unlikely that black English rules would ever allow for the production of words such as *ban'* (*bank*) and *buil'* (*built*) because of pairing of voiced and voiceless phonemes in the clusters.

Of particular importance is the manner in which these rules enter into the morphophonemic process. In the above examples, the clusters were integral parts of a single morpheme or base word, such as *chest*. The consonant cluster rule, however, also applies to the addition of bound morphemes /t/ and /d/ to free morphemes when there is no intrusive vowel. For example, *want* plus past tense gives *wanted*, creating a vowel–consonant final suffix. *Rob*, plus past tense, however, gives a final consonant cluster of *bd* and *stop* plus past tense gives a final consonant cluster of *pt*. In the two latter cases, the consonant cluster rule is functional because of the consonant–consonant combination and because both cluster phonemes are alike regarding voicing (*bd* contains two voiced phonemes, and *pt* contains two voiceless phonemes). In black English, therefore, *robbed* can be reduced to *rob'*, giving *He rob' the bank*, and *stopped* can be reduced to *stop'*, giving *She stop' the car*.

The plural formation as it pertains to the consonant cluster reduction rule provides further evidence of the consistency of black English. In standard English, when a word ending in a sibilant is pluralized it takes a suffix which phonologically approximates *iz*. The same rule holds forth for words such as *chest*, *mask*, and *test* that, when reduced in black English, are articulated as *ches'*, *mas'*, and *tes'*. As with standard English, these sibilant final words take the *iz* approximation as a plural suffix, giving *chesses* (*ches'* plus *iz*), *masses* (*mas'* plus *iz*), and *desses* (*des'* plus *iz*).

/r/ and /l/. Many of the previously mentioned researchers have noted that both /r/ and /l/ may be absent in the language of black English speakers. While the /r/ omission may occur in the language of white speakers throughout eastern New England, New York City, and parts of the South, it is frequently regarded as being even more common in the language of black English speakers in those geographic areas. Both /r/ and /l/ may be absent following a vowel, preceding a consonant, and between vowels. Fasold and Wolfram also have noted the apparent effect of these omissions upon grammar. For example, omission of /r/ in *their* removes the small phonologic difference between *they* and *their* allowing for the production of a sentence such as, *It is they book*. Omission of /l/ may affect the contracted form of *will* allowing for the production of a sentence such as, *He be going tomorrow*.

"-ing" suffix. The omission of the final /g/ in the *-ing* suffix is a common characteristic in the language of both standard and nonstandard speakers. A black English variation, however, is characterized by the absence of the entire suffix, giving *She is open the door*. Rather than representing a grammatical variation, Mc-David, Fasold and Wolfram, and others regard this as illustrative of the tendency among black English speakers to omit nasal consonants, in this case the *ng* sound.

/b/, /d/, and /g/. In black English, /b/, /d/, and /g/ are frequently substituted for by their voiceless cognates /p/, /t/, and /k/ when they occur in the final position of words and, occasionally, syllables. Such an occurrence allows for productions of *cap* for *cab*, *pat* for *pad*, and *tack* for *tag*. In some geographic areas, other voiced consonants undergo the same transformation.

A variation that may occur, which has significant importance for the morpho-phonemic process, is the tendency of some black English speakers to omit final /d/ and its voiceless cognate. Apart from the effect that this may have upon single-morpheme productions such as *bad*, giving *ba*, its importance in the production of past tense cannot be overlooked. The omission of either cognate can result in sentences such as *He stay here last night* and *She stop the car.*

QUESTIONS FOR DISCUSSION

1. What was the major problem in the design of the "language-deficit" studies?
2. What was unique about the design of the urban "language-difference" studies?
3. Which two professional organizations published position papers stating that no single dialect or language is more complex than another?
4. What was the landmark legal decision that recognized the validity of nonstandard dialects such as black English?
5. What is the purpose of bidialectal intervention programs?
6. What are two intervention alternatives apart from promoting bidialectalism?
7. Most intervention programs that promote bidialectalism are based upon what type of pedagogy?
8. What is included in the preparatory phase of bidialectal training?

REFERENCES

Adler S (1979). *Poverty children and their language.* Orlando, FL: Grune & Stratton

American Speech–Language–Hearing Association (1983). Position paper on social dialects. *ASHA, 25,* 23–24

Baskervill R (1977). The speech–language pathologist: A resource consultant for enhancing standard English competencies among inner-city children. *Language, Speech, and Hearing Services in Schools, 8,* 245–249

Blank M, & Solomon F (1969). How shall the disadvantaged child be taught? *Child Development, 40,* 47–61

Caplan S, & Ruble R (1964). A study of culturally imposed factors on school achievement in a metropolitan area. *Journal of Educational Research, 58,* 16–21

Cohn W (1959). On the language of lower-class children. *The School Review, 67,* 435–440

Fasold R, & Wolfram W (1972). Some linguistic features of Negro dialect. *Language, Speech and Hearing Services in Schools, 3,* 16–49

Feigenbaum I (1970). The use of nonstandard English in teaching standard. In R. Fasold & R. Shuy (Eds.), *Teaching Standard English in the Inner City* (pp 87–104). Washington, D.C.: Center for Applied Linguistics

Frentz T (1971). Children's comprehension of standard and Negro non-standard sentences. *Speech Monographs, 38,* 10–16

Johnson DR (1971). Should black children learn standard English? In M. Imhood (Ed.), *Social and educational insights into teaching standard English to speakers of other dialects* (pp 83–101). Bloomington, IN: Indiana University Press

Labov W (1975). *The study of nonstandard English.* Urbana, IL: National Council of Teachers of English

Linguistic Society of America (1972). Statement and resolution on language and intelligence. *Linguistic Society of America Bulletin*, March, 17–22

Loban W (1968). Teaching children who speak social class dialects. *Elementary English, 45*, 592–599

Martin Luther King Junior Elementary School Children v. Ann Arbor School District, 473 *F Supp*, 1371–1391 (E.D. Mich. 1979)

McDavid R (1970). On a hierarchy of values: The children of the dialectologist. In J. Akin et al. (Eds.), *Language Behavior* (pp 250–255). The Hague: Mouton Press

Ramsey I (1972). A comparison of first grade Negro dialect speakers' comprehension of standard English and Negro dialect. *Elementary English, 49*, 688–696

Stewart W (1964). *Nonstandard speech and the teaching of English.* Washington, D.C.: Center for Applied Linguistics

Williams F (1970). Some preliminaries and prospects. In F. Williams (Ed.), *Language and Poverty* (pp 1–10). Chicago: Markham Publishing Company

Wolfram W (1969). *Detroit Negro speech.* Washington D.C.: Center for Applied Linguistics

Wolfram W, & Fasold R (1974). *Social dialects in American English.* Englewood Cliffs, NJ: Prentice-Hall

10

Voice Disorders

Mary H. Pannbacker
Grace F. Middleton

EDITOR'S INTRODUCTION

Drs. Pannbacker and Middleton discuss the different voice problems manifested by young children and adolescents. These problems are frequently ignored by the classroom teacher; yet research has documented the need for appropriate identification and treatment of such disorders.

What should the teachers do? What are their responsibilities? These themes are of interest to the readers of this book and are addressed by the authors.

Mary Pannbacker has taught college and university courses in speech–language pathology for the past 21 years. Her major areas of interest and research have been cleft palate and diagnostic reporting.

Grace Middleton has taught courses in speech–language pathology at the university level for the past 20 years. Her research is concentrated primarily in the study of cleft palate, diagnostic report writing, and clinical supervision.

THE NORMAL AND ABNORMAL VOICE

Every voice is different with its individual characteristics easily identifiable by those who are familiar with the speaker. A voice is considered to be normal if it (1) is appropriate in pitch for the age, sex, and stature of the speaker; (2) is adequate in loudness for the speaking situation and is varied enough in pitch and loudness to be interesting, not monotonous; and (3) possesses appropriate quality: that is, is pleasant to listen to. Disorders of voice therefore are classified into abnormal pitch, loudness, and/or quality characteristics. These disorders occur in approximately 6–9 percent of the school age population. When academic and behavioral expectations are high and/or allergies and respiratory ailments are more prominent, the incidence may be higher.

ORAL COMMUNICATION PROBLEMS
IN CHILDREN AND ADOLESCENTS
Copyright © 1988 by Grune & Stratton, Inc.

A major problem faced by the school speech–language pathologist is early identification of children presenting voice disorders. The assistance of the classroom teacher is vital since many of these children are enrolled in regular classrooms and are functioning academically at grade level. When teachers do not recognize the symptoms of voice disorders, then the referral process tends to break down and the children do not receive needed services available to them.

Profile of School-Aged Voice-Disordered Child

In a 10-year review of voice-disordered children ranging in age from preschool through twelfth grade, Miller and Madison (1984) identified early twice as many voice problems in boys than in girls. They identified voice problems at all grade levels, but diagnosed more problems among children in preschool through grade five than in grades six through twelve.

Typically, the child who presents voice problems has a history of hoarseness and frequent episodes of upper respiratory infection or complications from allergies. Many of these children are talkative, vivacious, and outgoing. Others may be aggressive and loud. Those who scream and yell incessantly while on the playground are at high risk for voice disorders.

DISORDERS OF PITCH

The pitch of prepubescent children usually is perceived as somewhat high with little or no difference between boys and girls. During puberty, the pitch level of both girls and boys decreases or becomes lower. The larynx of the male between age 13 and 15 enlarges more rapidly and to a greater extent than that of females. The downward shift in pitch is therefore more dramatic in males.

During the pubertal changes in the larynx, the larynx is particularly vulnerable to abuse and misuse. Brand (1974, p 254) has pointed out that "during this period of muscular instability the voice should be kept free of strain, yet it is a time when vocal exertion tends to be at its greatest." Adolescents actively participate in sports or sit on the sidelines as enthusiastic spectators. They like to party in noisy and often smoke-filled areas.

Habitual pitch is the fundamental frequency most used by an individual speaker. An individual's optimal or natural pitch is the pitch that is most comfortable and easy to produce given the structure and function of that person's larynx. If there is a significant difference between one's habitual and one's optimal or natural pitch levels, then vocal problems are a likely result. Adolescents may try to convey a more mature image by speaking at a lower pitch than is comfortable. This is particularly true among boys trying to convey a masculine image. A lower fundamental frequency may be used in an effort to prevent embarrassing pitch breaks. Conversely, a functional falsetto production is characterized by continuing of preadolescent voice in postadolescent physically mature students. Some do not realize that they can use a lower pitch comfortably following the mutational changes. Others may be resistive of the change. Girls sometimes develop a high-pitched voice in an effort to convey a cute, vivacious image.

Too High or Too Low Pitch

Physical reasons for an unusually high pitch may include an anatomically small larynx for the person's age, sex, and stature; the presence of a congenital web located between the vocal folds; or laryngeal growth abnormalities of the vocal mechanism that may be related to endocrine disorders. Unusually low pitch may also be caused by endocrine disorders such as hypothyroidism, or by damage to those nerves that innervate the vocal folds. Low pitch may further be caused by the presence of vocal-fold pathology or formation of tumors within the masses of the vocal folds. Either high or low pitch may also be caused by learned behavior; for some psychological reason, the child or adolescent may use a higher or lower pitch than the optimum one that should be used.

Monotone Pitch

The monotone speaker drones on and on without energy or enthusiasm. Entertainers often capitalize on a monotone pitch and deadpan facial expression for a comedy effect. Lecturers, however, who use a monotonous pitch tend to bore listeners. Monotonous pitch may be related to a lack of precise neurologic control of laryngeal function, the presence of a hearing loss, or may be associated with emotional or personality factors.

Diplophonia and Pitch Breaks

Diplophonia refers to voice that sounds two-toned or having two different fundamental frequencies. Causal factors may include the presence of a pathology on the vocal folds or a breakdown in neurologic control of the muscles causing a unilateral vocal-fold paralysis. Breaks in pitch are involuntary pitch shifts often one octave in range. Pitch breaks may be ascending or descending in that pitch may shift an octave upward or an octave lower. We've all experienced pitch shifts during episodes of laryngitis when the vocal folds are swollen, or when we are under undue stress.

Another contributing factor may be voice change during puberty. In some adolescents, the voice changes are not completed, causing a high-pitched, weak, immature, and breathy sounding voice. The cause of this falsetto needs further investigation. Aronson (1985), however, theorizes that the etiology of this phenomenon is probably psychogenic immaturity, although there are plausible physical possibilities such as endocrine disorders, hearing loss, neurologic disorders, or lack of laryngeal activity during puberty due to a serious illness.

REFERRAL AND MANAGEMENT OF PITCH DISORDERS

Teacher

The teacher should refer a child presenting unusual pitch patterns to the speech–language pathologist. The speech–language pathologist may in turn refer the individual for a medical and/or psychological evaluation. If the child is enrolled in speech therapy, the speech–language pathologist must rely on the classroom teacher to serve as an important member of the management team. The teacher can help by observing carefully for any stress-related reactions of the child or situations that seem to cause pitch characteristics to change. Reducing the amount of stress on this particular child and observing the results could be of particular help in answering questions of etiology. The form in Figure 10-1 may be helpful to teachers in making referrals.

Speech-Language Pathologist

In therapy, the speech–language pathologist takes a case history from the child and the parents. The child is taught strategies for producing relaxed phonation, and pitch levels are manipulated in an effort to determine the child's optimal or natural pitch. Therapy may also include counseling the child with information relative to those parameters that convey an easy relaxed voice and possible reasons for use of a strained voice. The speech–language pathologist and the classroom teacher should keep each other informed about observations and programs in progress on a regular basis.

DISORDERS OF LOUDNESS

Loudness refers to the perceived intensity of voice. Optimal loudness is that which is appropriate to the environment and number of listeners. The voice should not be so weak that listeners cannot hear it, nor so loud that it irritates listeners and calls attention to itself.

Too Loud

The voice that is perceived by listeners as being too loud does not meet the criteria for normal loudness. Excessive loudness may be caused by the presence of a hearing loss, neurologic disorders, or may be related to emotional or personality factors. The use of excessive loudness is a form of vocal abuse that is often more typical among aggressive, dominant individuals. A common pattern found in some school-age children is the loud voice and aggressive personality.

TEACHER REFERRAL

TO: _____ Speech–Language Pathologist   RE: Disorder of Voice
      _____ School Nurse
Student's Name _____ Age _____ Sex _____
School _____ Grade _____
Teacher Making Referral _____ Room # _____

I am concerned about this student's voice because it
_____ sounds hoarse, rough or raspy
_____ sounds breathy or whispered
_____ sounds low-pitched when considering the age/sex of the child
_____ sounds high-pitched when considering the age/sex of the child
_____ sounds monotonous in pitch
_____ is too loud when considering environment and number of listeners
_____ is weak and difficult to hear
_____ is monotonous in loudness
_____ sounds hypernasal (talks through nose)
_____ sounds as if child's nose is congested

I am concerned with the following speech behaviors presented by this child:
_____ talks too fast   _____ uses long pauses
_____ talks a great deal   _____ is vocally very noisy
_____ talks too softly

I am concerned with the following nonspeech behaviors presented by this child:
_____ breathes through the mouth
_____ coughs frequently
_____ clears throat frequently
_____ laughs loudly and frequently
_____ appears to have problems hearing
_____ is frequently absent
_____ is easily angered
_____ has difficulty with peer relationships
_____ has frequent colds or upper respiratory infections
_____ has allergy problems

Factors Affecting the Child's Voice	Comment Below:	No Change	Better	Worse
Seasons	( )	_____	_____	_____
Time of day	( )	_____	_____	_____
Day of week	( )	_____	_____	_____
Weather	( )	_____	_____	_____
Emotional stress	( )	_____	_____	_____
Certain school activities	( )	_____	_____	_____
Certain people	( )	_____	_____	_____
Certain situations	( )	_____	_____	_____

Comments: (General behavior/adjustment, academic standing, family history, general
          health, other)

Fig. 10-1. Teacher Referral of a Voice Disorder

Too Weak

Inadequate loudness is characterized by a weak voice that makes it difficult for listeners to understand with ease. This pattern may also be associated with the presence of a hearing loss, lack of neurologic control of the laryngeal musculature, inadequate air pressure due to poor breath support, vocal-fold weakness caused by endocrine disorders, as well as emotional or personality factors including depression, low dominance, or poor self-esteem. It is this latter factor that is of particular importance in children; the weak or soft voice is frequently seen in youngsters who also manifest timid and shy personalities.

Monotonous Loudness

Monotonous loudness is characterized by a lack of variety in emphasis and stress patterns. Primary causes include neurologic, emotional, or personality factors.

REFERRAL AND MANAGEMENT OF LOUDNESS DISORDERS

Teacher

The teacher should refer the child who is perceived to speak too loudly, too softly, or at a monotonous loudness level to the speech–language pathologist (see Fig. 10-1). One of the first actions to be executed on the referral by the speech–language pathologist will be the administration of a test of the child's hearing sensitivity.

Speech–Language Pathologist

If hearing loss is ruled out as a cause of the loudness disorder, the speech–language pathologist may refer the child for a medical and/or psychological evaluation. Speech and language therapy usually includes the heightening of the child's awareness of what constitutes a loud versus a soft voice, the importance of an adequately loud but nonabusive loudness level, and the use of loudness variety to emphasize or stress important syllables, words, or phrases to convey meaning or emotion. Practice involving development of relaxed control of the child's breath support may also be appropriate.

Team Effort

Emotional or personality variables that affect loudness may be controlled through relaxation therapy and/or counseling in an effort to identify the underlying factors. Once the child can speak at an optimal loudness level, the classroom teacher may play a critical role in unobtrusively helping the child monitor and control loudness levels in the classroom setting. Often the teacher and child work out a signaling system so that undue attention is not called to the problem.

DISORDERS OF QUALITY

Voice quality problems can be divided into two categories: (1) *phonatory*, caused by laryngeal dysfunction and characterized by hoarseness, harshness, or breathiness, and (2) *resonance* that is either hypernasal or hyponasal.

Disorders of Phonation

It is essential that any person with a voice disorder be examined by a board certified laryngologist. Perkins (1977, p 174) pointed out that the speech–language pathologist ". . . may be the first to detect hoarseness, the early warning sign of laryngeal pathology: he knows that a patient's larynx, and perhaps his life, may hinge on referral to a physician for early detection of disease." More recently, Cohen, Geller, Thompson, and Birns (1983, p 437) in discussing voice change in infants and children, stated that "symptoms of dysphonia (weak voice) can be very early evidence of a serious problem, either within the larynx or resulting from a serious systemic disease." The phonatory disorders of harshness, breathiness, hoarseness, and vocal abuse–misuse, and their management will be discussed in this section.

There is a controversy about the terms used to describe phonatory voice disorders. The reason is probably that the terms mean different things to different listeners. For example, Boone (1977, p 43) stated "there is little agreement as to what these terms mean." What is hoarseness to one listener may be huskiness to another listener.

Harshness

Harshness is characterized by considerable tension and tightness during phonation and usually is described as an unpleasant, rough voice in which there are abrupt, harsh vocal attacks (sudden approximation of the vocal folds). It is often associated with an unusually low pitch (vocal or glottal fry) and/or inappropriate loudness levels.

The vocal or glottal fry usually is perceived as a bubbling, cracking type of low-pitch phonation and sounds like "popcorn popping." Harshness is almost always a functionally based (nonorganic) disorder of phonation, resulting from imitation, personality problems, or the use of inappropriate intensity and pitch levels.

Breathiness

Breathiness is characterized by a perceptible escape of unused air during phonation and sounds relatively weak or whispered. The vocal folds do not fully close and there is an audible escape of air. It is often associated with weak volume and/or low pitch.

Breathiness may be related to functional or organic etiologies. It may occur as a result of "poor vocal habits that result in improper breathing patterns and/or inefficient use of the larynx" (Polow & Kaplan, 1980, p 52). Breathiness is also considered a normal part of adolescence and precedes the change of voice. The organic causes of breathiness are related to either (1) diseases that inflame or swell the vocal folds and preclude approximation of the vocal folds or (2) neurologic deficits that adversely affect approximation of the vocal folds.

Hoarseness

Sometimes referred to as huskiness or roughness, hoarseness is a combination of harshness and breathiness, with the harsh element predominating in some hoarse voices and the breathy element in others. It is sometimes associated with unusually low or restricted pitch, pitch breaks, and/or intermittent aphonia (complete loss of voice or muteness). Hoarseness is very common and occurs at some time in almost everyone. It is sometimes overlooked and neglected because it often accompanies and subsides with a common cold. Hoarseness persisting for more than 10–14 days should not be ignored; the individual should be referred for an examination by a laryngologist.

Vocal Abuse/Misuse

Vocal abuse or poor vocal hygiene refers to vocal habits that have a traumatic effect on the vocal folds. Common types of vocal abuse include yelling, screaming, cheering, strained vocalizations, excessive talking, excessive throat clearing and coughing, inhalation of dust, cigarette smoke, or noxious gases, and talking in the presence of noise. Vocal misuse, the incorrect use of pitch or loudness, frequently coexists with vocal abuse and may cause chronic hoarseness.

Voice Management

Management of voice disorders is facilitated by a team of specialists working together. This team includes the laryngologist, the speech–language pathologist, the classroom teacher, and the parent. No one, child or adult, should begin voice therapy unless the larynx has been examined by a laryngologist and a voice evaluation has been done by a certified and trained speech–language pathologist.

Voice Therapy

Therapy for voice disorders is based on the findings of the laryngeal examination and the voice evaluation. Therapy usually is recommended if there is a significant voice problem that can be alleviated by elimination of vocal abuse and misuse. There are a variety of therapy techniques that may be used by speech–language pathologists to alleviate voice disorders. These techniques are used separately or in combination. The basic rule of application is to use the approach that works best. A number of approaches for eliminating or reducing harshness, breathiness, and hoarseness have been described in the literature (Aronson, 1980; Boone, 1977;

Case, 1984; Polow & Kaplan, 1980; Prater & Swift, 1984; Wilson, 1979, 1983; Wilson & Rice, 1977). Protective measures that are to be taken by the teacher to prevent abuse or misuse of their voice appear in the following list. The information has been adapted from Andrews and Shank (1983), Blonigen (1978), Polow and Kaplan 1980), Prater and Swift (1984), and Wilson (1979, 1983).

1. Be careful about using your voice at times when the larynx may be especially vulnerable; for example, when there is dryness or dust in the atmosphere or just before or during menstruation. Also, avoid talking when tense. Emotional tension may cause laryngeal strain and fatigue.
2. Stay away from dusty or smoky areas and limit the use of tobacco and alcohol.
3. Avoid shouting, screaming, yelling, cheering, fighting verbally, and excessive or loud talking.
4. Exercise regularly, but not too noisily or vigorously. Avoid talking when engaged in physical activity. Talk as little as possible when on a brisk walk or when jogging or running, especially when facing the wind.
5. Avoid excessive or loud coughing or throat clearing.
6. Do not make strange noises such as animal or machine noises. It is tempting to do this when reading stories to very young children.
7. Strive for easy, relaxed voice production. Speak with open relaxed throat and oral cavity. Speaking with tense closed restricted lip and clenched jaw movement increases laryngeal tension.
8. Avoid talking over excessive background noise, for example, when listening to loud music or riding noisy transportation, while others are talking loudly, or when around machinery.
9. Avoid talking when you have an upper respiratory infection such as a cold or when suffering from laryngitis.
10. Avoid using a loud whisper. A loud whisper places more stress on the vocal folds than does relaxed phonation and can cause inflammation of the vocal folds.
11. Be aware of vocal usage when acting in plays, singing, and giving speeches or oral reports.
12. Speak with adequate loudness for the situation and at an appropriate pitch and rate. Speak on the telephone at a normal conversational loudness level.
13. Avoid mouth breathing, especially in very cold weather.
14. Avoid certain foods and drinks before using your voice excessively or during episodes of hoarseness. Increased phlegm and accompanying throat clearing occurs after one has consumed dairy products (milk, ice cream, cottage cheese), chocolate, coffee or tea, brown colored sodas, or alcoholic beverages.

Prevention of Vocal Abuse in the Classroom

Classroom teachers can facilitate the reduction and elimination of vocal abuse in the classroom. It has been suggested that programs for prevention of vocal abuse should be instituted the day a child enters school and continue until past puberty.

The classroom teacher should give special attention to environmental quality that involves elimination and reduction of unnecessary noise in the classroom. It may also be appropriate to consider referring children who are facing stressful and disappointing experiences for assistance by a professional. Children should be given demonstrations of typical abuses by the classroom teacher or speech-language pathologist. Alternatives or nonabusive techniques should be provided such as pantomiming, whistling to call the dog or to attract a listener's attention, clapping rather than screaming at athletic events, walking across the street to talk to a friend instead of yelling, silent coughing and throat clearing instead of audible coughing and throat clearing, and walking away from machines that emit loud noises when one is conversing (Blonigen, 1978; Wilson, 1979).

The teenage years typically are active vocal years. This is a period characterized by frequent group activities, a heightened awareness of peer interactions, and frequent prolonged telephone conversations. Furthermore, teenagers are likely to engage in a variety of school and extracurricular activities that are vocally demanding and involve extensive use of the voice. Some of these activities, such as participation in athletics and cheerleading, usually do not provide voice conservation strategies.

Disorders of Resonance

Normal resonance is characterized by nasality for the production of the nasal consonants (m, n, ng). All other English speech sounds require oral rather than nasal resonance. Resonance disorders occur when there is any deviation in acceptable resonance, for example, deficient or totally lacking nasal resonance (hyponasality) to excessive nasal resonance (hypernasality). According to Peterson-Falzone (1982, p 527) hyponasality and hypernasality are frequently confused because of (1) "the traditional misinterpretation of the quality associated with a cold," and (2) "co-occurrence of hyponasality and hypernasality." The following sections cover the resonance disorders of hyponasality, hypernasality, and mixed nasality.

Hyponasality

Also referred to as denasality, hyponasality is the opposite of hypernasality. It results from the reduction in, or absence of, normal nasal resonance on the /m/, /n/, and /ng/. In the extreme form of hyponasality, /b/ is substituted for /m/, /d/ for /n/, and /g/ for /ng/. Hyponasality is frequently described as sounding like talking with a head cold or nasal congestion. An organic disorder for the most part, hyponasality results from some condition that occludes or obstructs the nasal passages or nasopharynx. Chronic hyponasality usually is caused by enlargement of the adenoid (pharyngeal tonsil). Due to the obstruction of the nasal airway, breathing through the mouth is common. Management of hyponasality involves medical identification and treatment of the obstruction responsible for this condition. Voice therapy is inappropriate.

Hypernasality

Hypernasality is characterized by too much nasal resonance, for example, sounds like talking through the nose. Assimilated or assimilation nasality is the least severe type of hypernasality and usually is not noticed by untrained listeners. It is characterized by excessive nasal resonance on vowels preceding or following the nasal consonants. Nasalized vowels are a more severe type of hypernasality than assimilation nasality. There is excessive nasal resonance on all vowels and glides /1/, /r/ regardless of the absence or presence of a nasal consonant. The most severe type of hypernasality is present on plosives /p/, /b/, /t/, /d/, /k/, /g/, fricatives /s/, /z/, /f/, /v/, /th/, /sh/, and affricatives /ch/, /j/ with or without hypernasality on vowels or glides.

Most, but not all, hypernasality is related to velopharyngeal incompetence, that is, coupling of the oral and nasal cavities so that airflow escapes nasally during production of nonnasal consonants. There are a number of conditions associated with velopharyngeal incompetence, such as (1) cleft palate; (2) structural abnormalities other than clefting, that is, submucous cleft palate (improper muscle attachment), congenital palatal incompetence (deep pharynx, short soft palate, and/or hard palate), or post adenoidectomy; and (3) paresis (weakness) from central or peripheral nerve damage. Although it is a rare condition, hypernasality may be present on a functional basis, that is, in the absence of any structural or neurologic disorder that could adversely affect velopharyngeal closure. There is, however, considerable evidence that functional hypernasality is probably marginal velopharyngeal incompetence and should never be considered functional.

Individuals who have hypernasality as a result of structural or neurologic impairment to the velopharyngeal mechanism usually have a variety of speech problems. In addition to hypernasality, these problems include defective articulation, nasal emission that is sometimes associated with facial grimacing, and phonatory voice disorders. Weak pressure consonants are associated with inadequate velopharyngeal closure that limits the ability to develop and maintain sufficient pressure in the oral cavity.

Nasal Air Emission

Nasal air emission is characterized by the escape of air from the nose during production of pressure consonants and is associated with inadequate velopharyngeal closure. Minimal nasal emission may be inaudible and does not affect sound production. Audible nasal emission affects sound production and is sometimes inappropriately referred to as "nasal snorting." Unusual facial postures, such as constriction of the nares or grimacing of the forehead and eyebrows, are frequently associated with nasal emission. These compensatory postures are attempts to prevent or reduce nasal emission and may be distracting.

Assessment of Velopharyngeal Function

Most speech–language pathologists use a variety of methods to assess velopharyngeal function, but the majority rely on noninstrumental techniques such as articulation testing, listener judgment, and oral examination. This is understandable since instrumental techniques are not readily available and are often rather expensive. The evaluation of velopharyngeal function must include instrumental assessment to confirm the presence of suspected velopharyngeal incompetence. McWilliams (1982, p 360) pointed out that to ignore instrumental assessment of velopharyngeal function "is to be guilty of malpractice and of administering speech therapy that may be inappropriate and even harmful and thus unethical."

Multidisciplinary Management

If velopharyngeal incompetence is suspected, it is necessary to recognize that referral for direct instrumental assessment of velopharyngeal function is needed. Radiography and/or endoscopy are the most frequently used instrumental techniques. Most cleft palate teams have the equipment necessary for such assessments. The 1986 Membership Team Directory of the American Cleft Palate Association lists 287 cleft palate teams in 48 states and the District of Columbia. These teams have plastic surgeons, prosthodontists, speech–language pathologists, and other specialists who can help determine whether or not surgical or prosthetic intervention is necessary.

Speech Therapy

Speech therapy alone will not remedy velopharyngeal incompetence. The interested reader may find discussions about the ineffectiveness of speech therapy for velopharyngeal incompetence elsewhere in the literature (McWilliams, et al., 1984; Rampp, et al., 1984; Ruscello, 1982). Failure to refer for physical management of velopharyngeal incompetence may result in delay of needed structural change as well as in compensatory vocal misuse (Cohn, et al., 1985).

ACKNOWLEDGEMENTS

Appreciation is extended to Wilma Jolley and Norma Frederick for reading the draft of this manuscript, to Jim Wilson for the illustrations, to Stella Camacho, Donna Halow, Alice Panko, Gina Venegas, Diane Wallace, and Margo Williams for their editorial assistance, and to Susan Moren and Rhonda Y. Washington for typing the manuscript.

APPENDIX A

Suggestions for the Classroom Teacher

1. Identify various voice problems more accurately by listening to audiotapes such as those developed by Aronson (1973), McWilliams and Philips (1979), and Wilson and Rice (1977).

2. Obtain publications about cleft palate by writing or calling the American Cleft Palate Educational Foundation, 331 Salk Hall, University of Pittsburgh, Pittsburgh, Pennsylvania, 15261; 800-24-CLEFT or in Pennsylvania 800-23-CLEFT.
3. Request information about communication disorders including voice problems from the National Association for Hearing and Speech Action, 10801 Rockville Pike, Rockville, Maryland, 20852; 800-638-8255, or in Alaska, Hawaii, and Maryland 301-897-8682 (collect).
4. Refer any child who is persistently hypernasal following cleft palate surgery or adenoidectomy to the speech–language pathologist for evaluation (see Fig. 10-1).
5. Contact the speech–language pathologist about any child who is scheduled for adenoidectomy so the child may be assessed preoperatively for any symptoms associated with velopharyngeal incompetence.
6. In cooperation with the speech-language pathologist, develop a preventive program with an emphasis on self-identification and self-monitoring of vocal abuse and misuse.

APPENDIX B

Anatomy and Physiology of the Vocal Mechanism

Larynx

Frequently referred to as the "voice box" by lay persons, the larynx contains nine cartilages that are held together by muscle, membranous and connective tissues. The larynx is located in the upper anterior part of the neck on top of the trachea and serves as the entrance to and protector of the breathing mechanism. Figure 10B-1 illustrates seven of the laryngeal cartilages from anterior and posterior views.

The thyroid cartilage looks like one of the fancier-shaped shields of a Roman soldier. The cricoid cartilage, which rests on top of the first tracheal ring, is circular and resembles a signet ring with the shank of the ring at the front of the structure and the larger signet portion at the back. At the top of the signet portion of the cricoid cartilage sit the two arytenoid cartilages. A three-dimensional view of these structures reminds one of the Egyptian pyramids, having three sides and three inferior corners called *processes*. The arytenoid cartilages are capable of rocking and sliding movements atop the signet portion of the cricoid cartilage. The small corniculate cartilages comprise the apices of the arytenoid cartilages.

The epiglottis is leaf-shaped and attaches inferiorly to the inside of the thyroid cartilage. The tip of the epiglottis can sometimes be seen at the root of the tongue in small children when the tongue is protruded and the mouth fully opened. The epiglottis serves to protect the larynx from runaway food particles during swallowing.

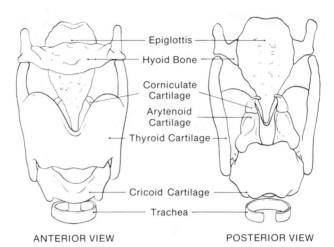

ANTERIOR VIEW   POSTERIOR VIEW

Fig. 10B-1. Anterior and posterior aspects of seven laryngeal cartilages.

Figure 10B-2 illustrates the location of the extrinsic muscles of the larynx that serve to elevate or lower the structure in the neck. Extrinsic muscles attach the larynx either to a structure located above it (such as the mandible [lower jaw] or the base of the skull) or to one located below it (such as the rib cage or the inside of the shoulder blade). Figure 10B-3 shows the intrinsic muscles that are self-contained within the larynx. These muscles serve to open and close the vocal folds and to

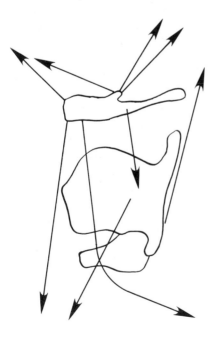

Fig. 10B-2. Schematic drawing of laryngeal movement facilitated by extrinsic laryngeal muscle activity.

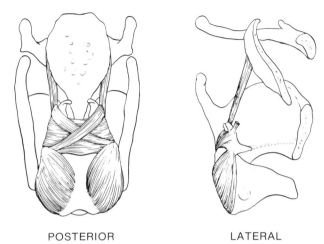

POSTERIOR   LATERAL
Fig. 10B-3.   Laryngeal musculature (posterior and lateral).

adjust the relationship between the thyroid and cricoid cartilages, thereby determining the individual characteristics of voice.

Figure 10B-4 illustrates the vocal folds, composed of two sets of intrinsic muscles running from the inside of the thyroid cartilage to the inside vocal processes of the arytenoid cartilages. Since the arytenoid cartilages are capable of rocking and sliding, the vocal folds are capable of opening and closing as illustrated in Figure 10B-4. The entire mechanism is finely timed and coordinated for voice production. Vocal fold pathology, neurologic dysfunction, hypertension in the mechanism, or any other cause for breakdown in the coordination of breathing and laryngeal function may cause abnormal voice production.

Velopharyngeal Function

The balance between oral and nasal resonance is determined by the "valving" of the soft palate or velum against the back of the throat or the pharynx. This valving activity is called *velopharyngeal function* or *closure*. The velum or soft palate is ele-

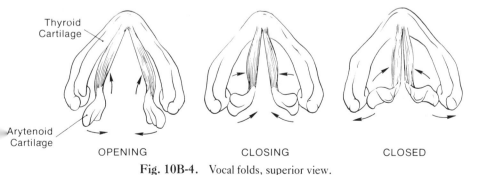

OPENING   CLOSING   CLOSED
Fig. 10B-4.   Vocal folds, superior view.

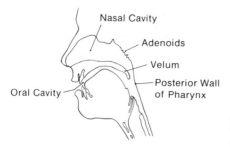

Fig. 10B-5. Lateral view of velopharyngeal mechanism.

vated symmetrically by the paired levator veli palatini muscles that originate on the temporal bone of the skull at the location of the Eustachian tube, and after coursing downward and forward, inserts in the middle third of the soft palate. When the paired levators work simultaneously and equally, the velum is elevated upward and pulled backward to valve against the pharyngeal wall. If one levator functions better than the other, then the velum moves asynchronously, and a gap or leak between the velum and the pharynx or throat is created, causing hypernasal resonance, that is, giving the impression to the listener that the speaker is talking through the nose. Additional causes of hypernasal resonance may include a velum that is too short to reach the posterior pharyngeal wall, a pharynx that is too deep for a normal-sized velum to reach, or impaired movement of the pharynx at the level of valving. Figure 10B-5 illustrates the primary structures that contribute to velopharyngeal function.

QUESTIONS FOR DISCUSSION

1. What characteristics constitute a normal voice?
2. Disorders of voice are classified under what three major areas?
3. List activities for preventing vocal abuse in the classroom.
4. Define vocal abuse and misuse and give examples of each.
5. What is the classroom teacher's responsibility in the prevention of vocal abuse and misuse?
6. Why is otolaryngological examination of the voice-disordered patient important?
7. Define velopharyngeal incompetence and give causal factors for this condition.
8. What is a cleft palate and how can this condition affect speech?
9. How do the classroom teacher and the speech–language pathologist coordinate their efforts in the management of disorders of voice?
10. Name the members of a cleft palate team.

REFERENCES

American Cleft Palate Association (ACPA) (1986). *Membership-team directory.* Pittsburgh: ACPA

Andrews M, & Shank K (1983). Some observations concerning the cheering behavior of school-girl cheerleaders. *Language, Speech, and Hearing Services in Schools, 14*, 150–156

Aronson AE (1973). *Psychogenic voice disorders.* Philadelphia: W.B. Saunders

Aronson AE (1980). *Clinical voice disorders.* New York: Thieme-Stratton

Aronson AE (1985). *Clinical voice disorders.* New York: Thieme-Stratton

Blonigen KA (1978). Management of vocal hoarseness caused by abuse: An approach. *Language, Speech, and Hearing Services in Schools, 9*, 142–150

Boone DR (1977). *The voice and voice therapy.* Englewood Cliffs, NJ: Prentice-Hall

Brand MN (1974). Childhood and adolescent dysphonias: The role of the speech teacher. *The Speech Teacher, 23* (1), 253–257

Case JL (1984). *Clinical management of voice disorders.* Rockville, MD: Aspen Systems

Cohen SR, Geller KA, Thompson JW, & Birns JW (1983). Voice change in the pediatric patient: Differential diagnosis. *Annals of Otology, Rhinology and Laryngology, 92*, 437–443

Cohn ER, McWilliams BJ, Garrett WS, Ferketic MM, Dressler BS, & Brown AF (1985). Pharyngeal flap surgery: Pre-operative and post-operative considerations for the speech–language pathologist. *Journal of Pennsylvania Speech and Hearing Association, 18*, 2–17

McWilliams BJ (1982). Cleft palate. In GH Shames & EH Wiig (Eds.), *Human communication disorders* (pp 330–369). Columbus, OH: Charles E. Merrill

McWilliams BJ, Morris H, & Shelton R (1984). *Cleft palate speech.* St. Louis: C.V. Mosby

McWilliams BJ, & Philips BJ (1979). *Audio seminars in speech pathology: Velopharyngeal incompetence.* Philadelphia: W.B. Saunders

Miller SQ, & Madison CL (1984). Public school voice clinics, part II: Diagnosis and recommendations—a ten-year review. *Language, Speech, and Hearing Services in Schools, 15* (1), 58–64

Perkins WH (1977). *Speech pathology: An applied behavior science.* St. Louis: C.V. Mosby

Peterson-Falzone S (1982). Resonance disorders in structural defects. In NJ Lass, LV McReynolds, JL Northern, & DE Yoder (Eds.), *Speech, language, and hearing: Volume II: Pathologies of speech and language* (pp 526–555). Philadelphia: W.B. Saunders

Polow NG, & Kaplan ED (1980). *Symptomatic voice therapy.* Tulsa: Modern Education Corporation

Prater RJ, & Swift RW (1984). *Manual of voice therapy.* Boston: Little Brown

Rampp DL, Pannbacker M, & Kinnegrew MC (1984). *VPI: Velopharyngeal incompetency.* Tulsa: Modern Education Corporation

Ruscello D (1982). A selected review of palatal training procedures. *Cleft Palate Journal, 19*, 181–193

Wilson DK (1979). *Voice problems of children.* Baltimore: Williams & Wilkins

Wilson DK (1983). Management of voice disorders in children and adolescents. *Seminars in Speech and Language, 4*, 245–258

Wilson F, & Rice M (1977). *A programmed approach to voice therapy.* Austin: Learning Concepts

11

Stuttering

Theodore Mandell

Editor's Introduction

Dr. Mandell introduces the teacher to a variety of tasks, methods, and goals that are helpful in relating to the stutterer. A therapeutic program is presented that can be implemented easily by the classroom teacher, hopefully with the guidance and support of the speech–language pathologist. The teacher should not utilize this information unless the speech–language pathologist concurs that such utilization is appropriate and desirable.

Dr. Mandell has worked with classroom teachers for many years. His chapter contains methods that have been used successfully by teachers in the Detroit Public Schools.

Stuttering can be defined succinctly as an abnormal disruption in the fluency or rhythm of speech.[*] Basically, there are two kinds of stuttering: primary and secondary.

PRIMARY STUTTERING

Primary stuttering is described as the easy, effortless repetition of sounds, syllables, words or phrases (M-m-m-Momma, may-may-may-I go out-go out and p-p-p-play?) *All* children go through such a stage of speech development, which is called *dysfluency.* Ordinarily, dysfluency occurs around the time when the child begins to speak in two-or three-word phrases and can disappear within weeks or months and, in some cases, years. Normal dysfluencies are rarely encountered after

---

[*] More specifically, there are two prevailing definitions of stuttering that have been adopted by most speech–language pathologists: (1) *Stuttering* is defined by the presence of certain specific disruptions in the speech pattern (i.e., repetitions and prolongations). (2) *Stuttering* is defined as a perceptual phenomenon as determined by observer agreements; that is, it is in the "ears" of the listener.

ORAL COMMUNICATION PROBLEMS
IN CHILDREN AND ADOLESCENTS
Copyright © 1988 by Grune & Stratton, Inc.

ISBN 0-8089-1887-7

the age of 6 or 7 years; abnormal dysfluencies gradually become more severe (some people call this transitional stuttering). As the children react even more negatively to the stuttering and manifest much fear and anxiety during their attempts to verbalize information, they enter the secondary stage of stuttering.

SECONDARY STUTTERING

Secondary stuttering is indeed a significant disorder. Speech is characterized by blocking spasms, usually on initial consonants or by prolongation and repetition of vowels ("B——ut I-ah-d—d—don't kn-kn-know the a——nswer." Secondary stuttering usually is accompanied by what are commonly labeled "secondary symptoms," for example, eye-blinking or bulging eyes, extraneous hand gestures, facial contortions, reddening of the face, head jerks or gasping for breath. These movements are part of the avoidance patterns that may make stuttering a bizarre disorder.

THEORIES OF CAUSATION

There are no certainties regarding the cause or causes of stuttering. But there *are* theories. A few are briefly discussed in the following paragraphs.

Emotional (Psycho-Sociopathic)

Some people believe that stuttering is a manifestation of a deep-seated personality (emotional, psychological) disorder. What is not known, however, is which is the cause and which is the effect. Is the stuttering a result of—or the cause of—the personality disorder?

Heredity

Research has shown that there is a higher incidence of stuttering in a stutterer's family history (which would include grandparents, parents, siblings, uncles, aunts, cousins) than in others. Thus, some people believe that this disorder can be genetically transmitted.

Developmental

The stutterer is normal in every respect *except* speech. It is believed by many people that stuttering is a learned behavior that develops out of the normal repetitive dysfluency and stresses of early childhood. External factors (i.e., overly concerned family members, mocking peers), however, may cause these children to feel worry, tension, and pressure. The children push themselves in order to produce the expected fluency, and the more they strain, the more they may block, thus developing into secondary stutterers.

Imitation

Relatively rare, but nevertheless real, is the case where individuals will become stutterers because they imitate one who is. Perhaps they notice that arrhythmic speech will allow for a minimum of class recitation, or that stutterers get a lot of sympathy, or they are not expected to become involved in communication. For them, stuttering is a nice, convenient escape. Parenthetically, stuttering acquired in this manner is most difficult to alleviate because most of the underlying bad habits or aberrations that many of the therapy systems attack are not present, and so the treatment is ineffective and the arrhythmic characteristics become ingrained.

Constitutional

The constitutional theory postulates that the nervous system of stutterers is incapable of handling the demands of communication made upon it, either because the auditory system cannot comprehend the speech signals received with the speed at which they are transmitted (they can't understand as fast as they hear), or because the oral musculature cannot move as rapidly as the brain demands.

BASIC ASSUMPTIONS AND OBSERVATIONS

Early environmental influences (such as parental reactions, frequent interruptions of speech, poor self-image) are important in determining whether a child's early dysfluencies are normal and will disappear, or eventually will evolve into secondary stuttering.

Secondary stutterers often tend to be more neurotic, more tense, more fearful, more introverted, and more psychologically unstable than nonstutterers. Adolescent stutterers are generally different from child stutterers. Sensitivity to dysfluency is greater; blocks are longer, stronger, more numerous; secondary symptoms are present; frustrations are more severe. Research consistently shows no relationships between IQ and stuttering, and four times as many boys stutter than girls.

GENERAL SUGGESTIONS FOR TEACHERS

Primary or Younger Stutterers

Teachers (and parents as well) *should not attempt* direct therapy,† that is, you should not give well-meaning advice ("slow down," "start again," "take it easy"). You should not overtly exhibit anxiety or concern. You should not comment on, criticize, or interrupt the speech of a stutterer. Despite some experimental programs in early

---

† It is assumed the speech–language pathologist will provide guidance to the teacher on the use of these techniques and suggestions.

treatment of beginning stutterers, this author believes that the best way to handle primary stutterers is to *ignore* their stuttering.

You *can* try to influence external factors: pressure or tensions in the classroom or home, sibling rivalry, bickering in the classroom or at the dinner table, inconsistent discipline in school or at home, unexplained disruptions of routine, insufficient rest or inadequate diet, unrealistic expectations or standards—*all of these can trigger primary stuttering spasms.* If you can effect a change in any of these factors, you could be of great help in alleviating this type of stuttering.‡

Specific Activities that Promote Fluent Speech

It is generally accepted that no stutterer stutters *all* the time. Therefore, observe the children to determine *when* they enjoy relative fluency and then exploit those periods. Give them maximum attention by getting them involved in oral activities that promote fluency.

Choral Speech

Both primary and secondary stutterers are far less dysfluent when they are reciting in and with a group. Therefore, have the entire class memorize a short poem or passage and then ask them to orally recite this passage. Every once in a while, through prearranged signs, have everyone stop except the row in which the stutterer is located. Further, and again on a prearranged signal, everyone in the row will stop except the stutterer. (The latter almost always will keep on talking, at least for a few words and will soon realize he or she *can* speak with fluency.) These procedures can be a part of the daily lesson plan, taking only a few minutes each day.

Rhyming Speech

Ask the stutterer, among others, to memorize small, very rhythmic poems ("Roses are red, violets are blue,") and then to recite them, first as a group, then individually.

Relaxation Drills

Have the entire group recite such poems as "Rag Doll," or "Jumping Jack Man," and accompany the words with the suggested body and muscle movements. Many of these poems can be found in children's books available in elementary school libraries.

Music in Unison

Rhythmic songs can be sung in unison periodically. Stutterers rarely suffer arrhythmia when singing rhythmic songs, even as individuals.

---

‡In a previous book, Sol Adler, *A Clinician's Guide to Stuttering,* C.C. Thomas, 1966, the editor has strongly supported such environmental manipulations. By eliminating or at least attenuating those factors that tend to enhance stuttering behavior, one can help to reduce the amount of stuttering manifested by the child.

Simon Says—a Variation

When you play this game, frequently change from an instruction for a muscle or limb placement or movement to an instruction for an oral production, or combine both. (Examples: Simon says, "Say, today is a 'sunny' day"; or Simon says, "Say, place your hands on your hips.")

Imitation

The teacher will state a phrase or short sentence slowly, using an easy, relaxed voice to "glide" or "slide" into the first utterance. Then, ask the stutterer to imitate this pattern, emphasizing the "easy" start and the slow rate. As the latter gains proficiency, the sentence length and rate of speech can be gradually increased until normal conversational patterns are achieved. This activity can be used either with a group of children or with the individual stutterer. The subject matter can be material the children are required to learn (spelling words, arithmetic concepts, reading drills). This kind of oral modification may extend the volitional control the stutterer possesses over speech patterns.

Gross Motor Speech Drills

Have the child toss a bean bag, and as it is released the child should recite a vowel, or a syllable, or one or more words. (This can also be a group activity.) Or, the child can bounce a rubber ball, and utter words or short phrases with each bounce-and-catch.

Stuttering Control Through Articulation Therapy

List the sounds and words on which the stutterer blocks. Then, instead of dealing with stuttering, the teacher instructs the child on the correct way of making the sound; for example, /p/ is difficult for many stutterers. Using the word *pie*, just touch the lips together lightly. First show them and then touch their lips, pressing them together gently and immediately after say *i;* the same can be done for the *b* in *bee* and the *t* in *two* and so on. By learning the correct mechanical productions, the child often progresses into more fluency with those sounds. For older children, the words can be incorporated into phrases or short sentences.

More Relaxation Drills§

Oral speech should emanate from a relaxed body as much as possible. Tension makes the muscles tighten and then soon grow tired. Relaxation loosens the muscles and rests them.

Goal. During speech, keep the muscles from becoming too tense and learn to relax these muscles at the proper rest pauses. The following exercises would be beneficial to *all* students—nonstutterers as well as stutterers:

---

§ A number of the following ideas were submitted to the author by different colleagues.

1. Stand erect, feet slightly apart. Drop head on chest. Then bend at waist, letting arms hang loosely. Raise trunk slowly until erect, then raise head.
2. Lower head to chest. Then begin to *slowly* roll head so that the ear reaches for a shoulder. Continue smooth, slow movement of head toward the back and complete circle to the other ear and finish with head on chest. Repeat several times.

Use of the Metronome

Set a regular piano metronome for 25–30 syllables (or 1-syllable words) per minute. This is truly slow motion speech. Ask the children to read from a word list or a nonsense syllable list in time with the beats. Again, watch the breathing and make sure they speak only on expiration and never on exhausted breath. "Blending" or "gliding" may be used here too; that is, while going from one word to another, continuous sound is maintained. Single words may be graduated into short phrases or sentences.

When fluency at the slow rate becomes routine, the metronome may be slowly increased until a conversational rate is ultimately reached. At any level, if difficulty is encountered (resumption of repetitions, hesitations, or blocks occurring too frequently), return to the slower rate. When fluency is relatively stable with this exercise, use a tape recorder so that on playback the children become their own positive role models. The goal is to maintain the achieved fluency after the metronome is turned off.

Hide and Seek (with Objects and Pictures)

Hide a few pictures (or toy models of the "real thing") of objects around the room that begin with the child's more difficult sounds, such as the plosives, dentals, or perhaps the sibilants. Ask the children to look for them and as they find each, they are to bring it to you or an appointed leader and identify what they have found. Stress proper breath pattern, slow rate, and continuous voicing between the article (a, an, the) and object. The entire class may be be involved in this activity.

Simultaneity of Speech and Writing (for Older Students)

Ask the students to go to the blackboard when you wish them to initiate a sentence or respond to a question. Make sure that they glide into the first sound and at the top of expiration. *Ask them to write as they speak* and not to stop at the end of each word, but instead connect each word—and do the same with their speech (i.e., Iwantabooktoread). Monitor the breathing and rate. If they stutter, they are to stop writing. When they are able to say a sentence fluently, ask them to step back, read it silently, turn around, visualize it, and then say it. If they block (and they have remembered to talk in full breath and glides), ask them to repeat the process.

Negative Practice (Homemade)

On strips of cardboard, paste pictures cut from old workbooks, readers, or magazines. On some of the cardboards paste a short original poem that can be completed by an obvious rhyming word. Ask the child to supply the word and repeat it three times.

> *Example* Cats scratch and birds sing.
> Dogs bark and bells _____ (ring, ring, ring).
> Mother cleans every room and sweeps the floor
> with a _____ (broom, broom, broom).

For those pictures without poems, ask the child to invent a simple but appropriate rhyming word. The pictures should be of familiar animals or objects.

> *Example* I have a cat
> It once caught a _____ (rat, rat, rat).
> *or*
> A yellow balloon
> Looks like the _____ (moon, moon, moon).

Modeling

The teacher organizes a set of pictures that show objects that can be named by a single word. The teacher goes through these cards one at a time, naming each one in a slow, relaxed but distinct manner and asks the child to repeat the word exactly the same way—slow, easy and relaxed, using the glide or slide into each beginning sound.

This one-word response level is continued for short periods during the following weeks until the child repeats easily and naturally the entire selection with confidence. Then, the teacher goes through the cards asking the child to identify them without the model, but in the same manner. When this is accomplished, short sentences and phrases may be modeled. For example, "This is a _____," or "We see the _____," may be repeated until, again, the modeling is omitted.

When the child's confidence level is high, more challenging aspects of the same activity can be developed. When a picture is held up, the child is asked to describe it or comment on it. From there, the activity may progress to talking about things in the room, first with modeling and then without. Finally, structured conversation might be attempted—like answers to questions. Again, this could be used with the whole class.

"Marked" Phrasing Drills (for Older Elementary Children)

Make sure that children can read, through review drills, short poems, and/or sentences. Then, via the chalkboard or on duplicated sheets of paper, indicate, by slash marks and/or symbols, where they, either individually or in unison, should pause, breathe (half or full breath), stop, raise or lower voice.

> *Example* "Roses are red / (half breath)
> Violets are blue / (half breath)
> Sugar is sweet / (half breath)

And so are you." (full breath)

or

"When I was a boy / I played baseball in
the summer / football in the fall / and
hockey in the winter." (full breath)

This can be a teacher's useful tool not only for helping stuttering children but also for reviewing a variety of lessons.

These activities are suggestions that can be used by classroom teachers for younger stutterers in the elementary range.

Secondary and Older Stutterers

At the beginning of this chapter, secondary stuttering was described as speech characterized by blocking spasms, usually on initial consonants, or by prolongation or repetition of, or hesitation on vowels, and usually is accompanied by extraneous secondary symptoms such as hand gestures, foot stamping, and facial contortions. Secondary stuttering often emerges from the improper handling of primary stuttering. Onset of secondary stuttering very often can also occur right after personal trauma (death of a family member, sudden fright or shock, injuries).

Direct intervention by such techniques as classroom activities occurs less frequently with secondary stutterers. (1) The children are older and the stuttering is more severe and rigid and less amenable to intervention within their peer group and by someone not trained as a speech pathologist. (2) The classes are larger and more impersonal, and instructional activities and techniques are not suitable. There are indirect ways, however, in which the teacher can be of tremendous supportive help.

1. Be a good, smart listener. Let the stutterers, whether they are reciting in class or talking to you, always finish their statements. Don't interrupt them or supply words for them. If possible, when the students are out of the room, educate the rest of the class to control their reactions. Look the stutterers right in the eye and never break eye contact. This tells them you're interested, you care about *what* they are saying and not *how* they are saying it.

2. Help stutterers accept themselves as stutterers. Stuttering is something they *do*, not something they *are*. Again, try to educate their peers. Just as eyeglasses help vision and hearing aids help hearing, and they are accepted as natural phenomena, so can controlled reactions to the stutterers' speech help them by not making them self-conscious, embarrassed, or ashamed.

3. Help the stutterers understand that there are gains they may have to relinquish if they learn to control their stuttering. That is to say, they will no longer be able to use their stuttering as a crutch, and they will have to recite just like everyone else, and, likewise, accept the same responsibilities as everyone else.

Goals for the Teacher

The following is a list of goals for the teacher–stutterer relationship:

1. Eliminate or reduce the tensions and pressures with which the stuttering could be associated, that is, (1) as much as is possible, be sure that the demands placed on stutterers are understood and are reasonable; (2) let them know in advance whether they will be called on for oral recitation; (3) make sure your discipline is consistent; (4) try to insure a calm environment (keep peer group pressures in the classroom, at least, to a minimum); and (5) try to be aware of any causes for their nervousness or insecurity in your classroom and reduce them.

2. *Eliminate secondary symptoms.* Privately tell them that you don't mind them stuttering when they recite—"You can relax about your feelings about your blocking in the classroom, but see if you can do it without extraneous eye-blinking or gestures."

3. *Modify the block.* Again, privately remind them that if they feel they are going to block while speaking, they should try to alter their stutter. Instead of a "stop-block," that is "B————ut there's a d—ifferent answer," they should "bounce" it, that is "Bu-bu-but there's a di-di-di-different answer."

4. *Modify faulty habits.* Arrange a series of signals between you and them so that if they are talking on exhausted breath, you'll touch your nose, or if they are talking too fast, you'll tug at your ear.

5. *Improper phrasing.* It is appropriate to drill the class via the "slash /" technique when reciting, that is, have the class recite in unison some passage where you have indicated the appropriate places to pause via the "slash /," and when the stutterers are reciting, use an appropriate silent signal prearranged between you and them when they are violating that rule.

6. *Excessive tensions of the speech mechanism.* A brief conversation (couple of minutes) before class with the stutterers won't hurt to remind them that if they recite in this hour, they should remember to use a relaxation technique of rolling their head or "dropping" it to relax their neck muscles, and deep breathing to relax the thorax and abdominal muscles.

7. Note what situations in which they are more apt to stutter than others and try to avoid or minimize them, that is, do they stutter more right after lunch, or at the beginning of class, or before or after a specific subject? If so, avoid calling on them at these times.

8. If there is to be recitation by a number of students, inform the stutterers beforehand when you're going to call them or even let them know what you're going to ask them to do without telling them the answers. This sounds as if you are giving them an unfair advantage but the author prefers to think that you are giving them an even break.

9. Promote recitative situations when the stutterers appear to be particularly fluent. For example, ask them to read poetry or other rhythmical material, or to

recite material that has been previously prepared with slash and breathing signals; or have them recite while at the chalkboard and demonstrate what they are talking about. This allows them to coordinate large and small muscle movement with speech and may help to distract them from the fear of blocking.

A Final Reminder

Direct therapy by the classroom teacher is difficult. Even if you know what to do, or can be trained to do it, *you just don't have the time*. The information presented in this chapter may therefore be of limited value to you and to your arrhythmic students. Hopefully, however, what you have read will help to reduce the uncertainties and fears you may hold when confronted by the phenomenon called stuttering. Finally, establishing two-way communication between yourself and the speech–language pathologist is vital. Your knowledge of the child, the home environment and the classroom environment, coupled with the speech–language pathologist's expertise, can form a powerful team in the struggle to help the stutterer overcome the problem.

APPENDIX: A SUMMARY STATEMENT

Dos and Don'ts for the Teacher of Young Stutterers

1. Do not label the children as stutterers; initiate a conversation with them as soon as possible and ascertain if they consider themselves stutterers.
2. Have they been (or are they) receiving speech therapy? If so, what is the status of the therapy? If not, contact your public school speech–language pathologist.
3. Do all you can to enhance their self-concept; make them feel good about themselves by lavishing praise upon them.
4. See to it that no one pokes fun at them or imitates their stuttering. Many years ago, for example, we found a ten year old girl being severely hassled on the bus ride to and from school. Our communication with the school principal and bus driver soon put an end to this behavior.
5. No one should offer any well meant but useless advice such as "think before you talk." Such advice often escalates the problem rather than helps the children.
6. Watch their faces as they talk and do not indicate any impatience.
7. Along with the speech–language pathologist and parent, try to foster an environment for them that on the one hand is devoid of many pressures and negative expectations, and on the other hand enhances the frequency of speaking situations that encourage fluency.
8. A concerted plan of action should be initiated involving all the adults who interact with the stutterers, that is the speech–language pathologist, teacher, and parents.

QUESTIONS FOR DISCUSSION

1. What is a simple definition of stuttering?
2. What are the differences between primary and secondary stuttering?
3. Describe at least two theories of the cause of stutteing.
4. Describe two activities to be used by the classroom teacher for stutterers.
5. What are some nondirect activities the teacher can use for secondary stutterers?
6. What is at least one basic assumption to be made regarding stutterers?
7. Most stutterers do not stutter *all* the time. They *do* have periods of relative fluency. Of what significance is this to the classroom teacher?
8. How do you work with stutterers through articulation therapy, and why?
9. Why is relaxation so important for the stutterer?
10. What are some of the external factors that may aggravate stuttering?

RECOMMENDED READINGS

The following general readings are suggested to those teachers who are desirous of obtaining additional information concerning this disorder. Your speech–language pathologist should be able to recommend other books or articles specific to your needs.

Ainsworth S (1975). *Stuttering: What it is and what to do about it.* Lincoln, NE: Cliff Notes, Inc.

Bloodstein O (1975). *A handbook on stuttering.* Chicago: National Easter Seal Society for Crippled Children and Adults

Speech Foundation of America, (1966). For Titles of Publications Relevant to Stuttering, write to P.O. Box 11749, Memphis, TN

Van Riper C (1973). *The treatment of stuttering.* Englewood Cliffs, NJ: Prentice-Hall

Van Riper C (1982). *The nature of stuttering* (2nd ed.). Englewood Cliffs, NJ: Prentice-Hall

12

Articulation

Rhonda S. Work

EDITOR'S INTRODUCTION

Articulation disorders are the most common of all oral communication disorders, and there is much teachers can and should be doing to ameliorate these problems in their classrooms. In her capacity as a Program Specialist Supervisor, Rhonda Work has acquired extensive practical information that will be helpful to the classroom teacher. This chapter reflects her awareness of teachers' needs vis-à-vis childhood articulation disorders.

Daniel Webster said, " . . . if all my possessions were taken from me with one exception, I would choose to keep the power of communication, for by it I would regain all the rest." Mr. Webster truly understood that to express oneself easily and effectively is one of the most fundamental, personal aspects of life. Without this ability children may be seriously handicapped in their social, emotional, and educational life. Documentation shows that both speech and language follow a normal, sequential pattern of development (Sander, 1972; Templin, 1957). It has been demonstrated, however, that not all children develop efficiency and accuracy of speech sound production at the same time (Hodson & Paden, 1983; Van Riper, 1972). In fact, correct production of some sounds and sound combinations may not be expected until after the child has reached 5–8 years of age. But how often we expect clear, distinct speech from kindergarten and first grade children!

Table 12-1, based on Templin (1957) and Berry and Eisenson (1956), is a representation of normal speech development. Although the information in Table 12-1 is based on data that are thirty years old, there have been no newer studies to contradict these earlier findings. Therefore, even a brief study of Table 12-1 suggests that speech sounds develop at different rates for different ages. This information is very useful when helping parents understand their child's speech production skills in relation to normal speech development.

Perhaps the reader is wondering what speech has to do with articulation disorders, the topic of this chapter. A few definitions at this point may be helpful. *Speech*

ORAL COMMUNICATION PROBLEMS
IN CHILDREN AND ADOLESCENTS
Copyright © 1988 by Grune & Stratton, Inc.

Table 12-1
An Easy Guide to Normal Speech Development in Children*

3	4	5	6	7
Boys				
p	ng	y	zh	f
b			wh	l
m			j	r
h				ch
w				sh
d				s
n				z
k				th (voiceless)
t				v
g				th (voiced)
Girls				
p	l	j	sh	s
b	t	y	ch	z
m			r	th (voiceless)
w			zh	v
d		f	f	th (voiced)
n			wh	
k				
g				
h				
ng				

Source: Based on Templin M (1957). *Certain language skills in children.* Minneapolis, MN: University of Minnesota Press, and Berry M, & Eisenson J
(1956). *Speech disorders: Principles and practices of therapy.* New York:
Appleton-Century-Crofts, Inc.
Note: Consonant blends—tr, bl, pr, etc., develop between ages 7–9.
*Age at which 90% of boys and girls can articulate sounds. Vowel sounds
are produced correctly by 90% of all children by age three.

is the audible motor production of sounds and sound patterns and includes adequate
voice quality and rhythm. *Articulation,* as defined by Phillips (1975, p. 36) "is the
process of forming meaningful oral symbols by the manipulation of the articulators—
the tongue, lips, lower jaw, teeth, and soft palate." A more recent concept in
speech–language pathology has been to include articulation in the term phonology.
Phonology is considered the sound structure of language and has two components, "a
systematic repertoire of meaningful sounds (phonemes) and a finite set of rules
defining how these phonemes can be arranged sequentially" (Hodson & Paden,
1983, p. 2). In other words, phonology is not only the sounds of the language, but
also the rules that tell us how we can use these sounds. For the purposes of this
chapter, we will use the term articulation with the understanding that it encompasses

the definitions cited above for speech, articulation, and phonology. With this in mind, let us examine articulation and the prevention of articulation disorders.

THE PREVENTION OF ARTICULATION DISORDERS

Normal Articulation Development

As Table 12-1 demonstrates, there is a specific sequence of speech sound development. Those sounds that are learned earliest are sounds that are easier to make, such as /p/, /b/, /t/, or /k/. Other sounds that require more discrete movement of the articulators are learned at a later age. For example, the most commonly misarticulated sounds, /s/, /l/, /r/, and /th/, are not expected to be perfected by all children until ages seven or eight. This is not to say that many children may learn to say these sounds before age eight, but for those children who still are learning /s/ or /r/ or /l/ or /th/, we should not become overly concerned until first, second, or even third grade. This approach may apply also to the use of certain consonant blends, such as /str/, /gr/, or /fl/. The school speech–language pathologist is trained to identify children who may not be using one of these sounds (as well as any other sounds) and to determine which children should be enrolled in speech therapy.

Factors Related to Articulation Development

The ability to articulate clearly and effectively is dependent on several factors. Of greatest impact is the age of the child. As may be surmised by the foregoing discussion of Table 12-1, age has a great deal to do with the development of articulation. We would accept certain sound production from a 3 year old, but would find that same production unacceptable in a 7 year old. A 7 year old who is still saying "titty tat" for "kitty cat" would most certainly draw attention to the speech pattern and might even be ridiculed by classmates. We would be much more tolerant of a 3 year old saying "titty tat," although we might expect correct use of the /k/ sound on an intermittent basis, as three is the age at which /k/ is produced by most children. Thus, the acquisition of sounds is linked to the age of the child.

A second factor influencing the development of articulation is the physical and structural development of the articulators: the tongue, teeth, lips, jaw, and soft palate. The vast majority of children develop normal articulation patterns because there is little or no malformation of the articulators. Even with minor deviations, such as poorly aligned teeth or a short upper lip, children compensate and learn to use the speech sounds adequately. There are those children who have serious physical handicaps and who require speech therapy to learn to approximate the production of certain speech sounds. The child with a cleft palate or with cerebral palsy must compensate for a structural difference and, therefore, benefits from speech therapy by learning alternate ways to say sounds. With new technology for physical repair and for alternate methods of communication, the damage done by structural deviations is being mitigated so that children with the most severe physical handicaps can learn to communicate.

For children to be able to say the sounds of their language, they must be able to hear and to listen, but we must remember that there is a difference between hearing and listening. *Hearing* refers to the physical ability to receive sound, while *listening* encompasses the more complex process of sorting sounds and putting meaning to sound. Since listening plays such an important role in sound production, helping children to listen correctly is of utmost importance. Equally important is the learning of sound discrimination, sound blending, and sound integration. It would appear that the development of articulation is based in large part on appropriate listening.

Intelligence has been found to be a factor related to articulation development, although not as significantly as might be expected. In fact, articulatory efficiency and intelligence are not closely correlated except at the lower range of intelligence. Studies have shown that individuals with IQs below 70 have more articulation disorders than people with normal or above normal IQs. This may be due to the individual's inability to adequately understand and apply the rules of phonology, which is a cognitive function. Whatever the reason, more patience and acceptance is needed when listening to the child who is mentally handicapped and who has an articulation disorder.

These four factors, then, have a relationship to the development of articulatory skills. When considering children's articulation or speech sound production, we must also consider their age, physical development, hearing and listening skills, and cognitive ability.

Prevention and Speech Improvement

Perhaps the single most important approach to articulation disorders is the prevention of these disorders. Much should be done prior to the child's entering school, but even after enrollment in kindergarten, children will respond positively to speech improvement activities.

Practically speaking, children enter school with many different backgrounds and experiences. These experiences may or may not have prepared them for the world of learning. As a result, every teacher can relate the difficulties and the challenges encountered when a new class of students walks through the classroom door. Even though the first five years of a child's life are considered to encompass the optimal period for speech and language growth, entry into school does not preclude the need for continued growth in communication skills. The amount and degree of speech stimulation in the classroom will shape students' speech and language growth. Teachers are in the unique position to serve as good role models, to provide stimulation of sound, to reinforce correct sound production, and to offer the children many opportunities to explore their world and the world of sound.

Evidence that speech improvement is a prevention tool for academic learning has been demonstrated in several studies. Research by Sommers et al. (1961)

suggested that reading scores can be raised when children receive speech training. Evaluation of a speech improvement program conducted in first and second grade revealed that a coordinated speech improvement program significantly improved articulation skills of many of the children, that the children demonstrated a new interest in speaking and listening skills, and that the program supplemented and strengthened the phonic skills program (Work, 1968). Speech science research has provided information about vocabulary use and the ability to auditorially discriminate sounds (Stark & Wallach, 1980) and the linkage between phonology and reading (Atkinson & Canter, 1979; Liberman, Shankweiler, Camp, Heifetz, & Werfelman, 1977).

It becomes apparent, then, that speech improvement has a role to play in the development not only of speech and language skills, but also of the academic learning process. By enhancing the children's growth in speech, we can enhance the opportunities for growth in learning. A well-planned speech improvement program integrated into the curriculum can provide for better speech and better learning.

TYPES OF ARTICULATION DISORDERS AND THEIR CAUSES

Types

It is not surprising that children with speech and language disorders make up the largest group of students in exceptional student programs. It has been estimated that nearly half of these children have articulation problems. What is an articulation disorder? Articulation is considered defective when speech sound production contains substitutions, distortions, omissions, or additions of sounds in a manner that is not commonly acceptable to the listener.* A common example of misarticulated sounds is found in baby talk, a form of developing speech through which most children progress on their way to adult speech. Frequently, one hears "tootie" for "cookie" or "pay" for "play." These speech patterns are part of the developmental process and should not be considered deviant unless found in older children. There are, however, some markers that can aid in a better understanding of articulation disorders.

Substitutions

Perhaps the most common type of articulation disorder, substitutions, may be defined as the use of an incorrect sound or a different sound for the one intended for use. The types of substitutions frequently heard in the classroom include /w/ for /r/ as in "wabbit" for "rabbit," or /th/ for /s/ as in "thun" for "sun," or /w/ for /l/ as in "wamp" for "lamp." The most frequently misarticulated sound is /s/ and its most

---

*The articulatory patterns produced by social dialect speakers as a function of their sociolinguistic environment should not be considered defective. This matter is discussed by Dr. Bountress in Chapter 9.

frequent mode of misarticulation is the lisp. A lisp is characterized by /th/ for /s/, and, in most cases, follows a developmental pattern. In fact, most substitutions are predictable, although there is always an exception to the rule.

An important consideration to keep in mind when observing a student using substitutions is the expected age of development of the misarticulated sound. Referring to Table 12-1 again, a child who is 5½ years old and lisping may still be in the maturational process of learning to produce /s/ correctly. On the other hand, if that same child is substituting /t/ for /k/, we might safely say that there is an articulation problem. As stated earlier, the speech–language pathologist can assist in the determination of such a problem.

Omissions

Omissions usually are found in the speech of very young children. This is not normally a problem, as it is part of the process of learning new sounds. Omissions in young children occur most frequently at the end of words, such as "ba" for "ball." As children learn new words, the sounds become part of the repertoire of speech production. When a child persists in omitting sounds beyond expected learning levels, the intelligibility for the listener decreases and an articulation problem emerges. A rule of thumb is that omissions should not occur in the speech of school-age children except for some consonant blends. Certainly by third grade or age nine children should be using all sounds in all places.

Distortions

When a sound is made that approximates the correct sound but is slightly different, it may be viewed as distorted. A common distortion is the lateral or "slushy" /s/ where the sound escapes over the sides of the tongue instead of the tip of the tongue as it is placed behind the teeth. Distortions are more frequently found in older children, follow a pattern, are persistent, and may be very difficult to correct. Another form of distortion is noted when vowel sounds are not pronounced correctly. Although this is a less frequent occurrence, it, too, is a difficult problem for correction. It appears that auditory discrimination plays a role in the inability to correctly produce distorted sounds, for the distortion when compared to the correct sound may be so minimally different that any lessening of auditory discrimination would impede the understanding of the sound differences.

Additions

Additions are the least frequently occurring misarticulations and often are linked to regional dialects. We are familiar with the Boston "Cuber" for "Cuba" and would not consider this an articulation disorder. There are, however, some individuals who add a sound to a word, like "prentzel" for "pretzel," or who insert "uh" at the end of words in conversational speech. These additions may cause the speech to

be considered defective when they interfere with the intelligibility of the communication. Speech therapy can be successful in modifying distortions or eliminating
additions that occur in the speech of an individual.

Causes

As so often is true in any behavior that is different from the norm, causation
may be difficult to pinpoint. In the case of articulation disorders, it is felt that most
problems are functional in nature, that is, there is no organic or sociolinguistic cause
of the disorder. Functional articulation problems appear to be the result of faulty
learning or faulty listening. For some reason the child has persisted in using faulty
speech patterns beyond the age expected for correct use of the sounds. This may be
due to poor speech models in the home where one of the parents or an older sibling
has the same speech pattern. Or it may be due to a poor understanding of the rules
of phonology, rules that normally are learned naturally but may have to be taught to
certain children. Or it may be due to a lack of stimulation or motivation. No matter
what the functional cause, it is important to provide the motivation, the stimulation,
and a good role model in the classroom.

Some articulation disorders are organically based. Children born with cleft lips
or palates will have difficulty producing speech sounds if early physical repair is not
provided. Even with surgical intervention prior to the onset of speech, some residual
difficulty may be expected, such as a shortened upper lip that prohibits good
articulation of the plosive sounds /p/ and /b/ or some minimal nasality due to poor
closure of the passages to the nasal cavities. Usually, approximations and modifications can be taught so that the adverse effects of these problems can be reduced.

Another organic articulation problem is one related to cerebral palsy. Cerebral
palsy is manifested in poor muscle control throughout the body, and those muscles
necessary for the production of speech sounds are certainly involved. The muscles
may be either too lax or too taut with accompanying poor breath control and
excessive head and body movement. Speech therapy for children with cerebral
palsy provides assistance in learning to control some of the muscle movement or to
find acceptable approximations for selected speech sounds. With the advent of the
computer age, many cerebral-palsied students have found a new avenue for communication through assistive learning devices, communication boards, and computer-
enhanced speech.

For any child with a physical impairment such as cleft lip/palate or cerebral
palsy, a problem usually as serious as a speech disorder is that of acceptance by
school peers. The classroom teacher has a splendid opportunity to set the tone for
both understanding and acceptance of the child's handicap and the child's speech
disorder.

Articulation problems have been linked to other factors such as mental retardation, emotional disturbance, or personality disorders. As discussed earlier in this
chapter, individuals whose intelligence is at the lower end of the scale have been
found to have more articulation problems than individuals with higher IQs. We must

be cautious and not assume that all mentally handicapped children have articulation disorders, for there are those children with reduced cognitive ability who do have command of acceptable speech patterns. Conversely, a child who has a severe articulation disorder with no apparent physical handicap should not be viewed as retarded. There could be any number of reasons, as already described that make speech unintelligible. Once again the teacher can be the role model for understanding, acceptance, and good speech.

Research has suggested that unstable homes or families with emotional problems have a higher proportion of children with articulation disorders. This may be due to lack of consistency in positive family relationships or to the inability to accept the child's speech, perhaps even ridiculing it. A lack of acceptance can produce frustration and anxiety for the child and can lead to continuing problems, including a poor self-image. In such cases, it would be helpful if professionals from several different areas of expertise collaborate on the best course for the treatment.

The Language Link

As educators have become more knowledgeable about language, the relationship of articulation defects to linguistic disorders has been investigated. As early as 1969, Shriner, Holloway, and Daniloff concluded that children with articulation problems used shorter sentences and more immature grammatical structure. Whitacre, Luper, and Pollio (1970) also found that knowledge of phonologic and grammatical rules was less accurately understood and used by children with articulation disorders as compared to peers without articulation problems. In his research in 1974, Panagos found that children with severe articulatory deficits also had problems with syntax and semantics. Finally, Ingram (1976) concluded that children with severe articulation problems exhibited a language disorder of a phonologic type, that is, a problem in both sound production and the application of the rules of the sound system, rather than a problem of a phonetic type of the inability to produce correct sounds.

To summarize, the various types of articulation disorders may be the result of faulty learning, organic abnormalities, or emotional problems.† There is a need to understand the cause whenever possible and to provide an atmosphere of support and acceptance. Recognition of the link between articulation and language will provide a framework for developing successful speech activities.

TREATMENT PROGRAMS

Speech–language pathologists have been trained to remediate a variety of speech and language disorders. In designing therapy for articulation disorders, sev-

---

†Other but less common causes are hearing loss and inappropriate swallowing behavior—better known as tongue thrusting.

eral approaches based on a particular rationale have been developed. In most cases, these approaches have similarities as well as differences. The major goal of any treatment program is to achieve correct, or as near correct as possible, production of the speech sounds in all linguistic environments. The objectives or techniques to reach this goal may vary, but the goal remains the same. For those students with functional articulation disorders, correct production should be achievable unless some emotional barrier exists to prevent success. For students with organically based articulation disorders, an acceptable approximation of speech sounds may be all that can be achieved; thus improvement in sound production is the goal.

Early Theories and their Applications

As early as 1927, Scripture and Jackson published a manual outlining for the first time in a systematic manner a program for articulation therapy. Their major emphasis was on instructing the student in phonetic placement techniques, breathing, relaxation, and "mouth gymnastics." The gymnastics were a set of exercises for the articulators done in preparation for learning to place the articulators in the correct positions for appropriate sound production. An extension of the gymnastics technique was provided by Stinchfield-Hawk and Young in 1938 when they introduced the *motokinesthetic method*. This method stressed the need to develop the speech muscles through stimulation or manipulation so that the student would understand how the articulators worked to produce sound. Both of these approaches stressed correct placement of the articulators for the correct production of speech sounds.

Van Riper first reported his method in 1939 and included steps that highlighted motoric and acoustic aspects of sound production. His program went beyond phonetic placement techniques, however, and included the need for the student to hear, identify, and compare correct and incorrect use of a sound. These ear training techniques became the basis for the therapy program, since the student always is expected to listen and compare as the progression through single word, syllable, phrase, sentence, and conversational speech is achieved.

A shift away from motor sound production became apparent when Backus and Beasley (1951) introduced a type of psychotherapeutic approach to articulation therapy. They emphasized the need for group, not individual, therapy to provide for modeling of the correct sound by the speech–language pathologist or another member of the group. Rather than direct therapy techniques, Backus and Beasley relied on group dynamics and directive counseling to assist students in the development of correct sound usage.

Also in 1951, Jakobson, Fant, and Halle developed the *distinctive feature theory*. This theory classifies sounds according to the manner and place of articulation and, more importantly, identifies the sounds according to their minimal contrastive sound units. The authors listed features such as consonantal/nonconsonantal, voiced/ voiceless, and nasal/oral, to name just three of the ten pairs of language features.

Recent Theories and their Applications

Sommers and Kane (1974), using the distinctive feature theory, reported on the *wedge approach* to therapy whereby sounds that share distinctive features and are misarticulated by the student are selected for therapeutic intervention, but only one of the sounds is actually targeted for correction. The idea is that by correcting one sound, the other sounds in that group will improve because of generalization.

A most recent entry into the field of treatment theories is that of the *phonologic approach* to the remediation of articulation disorders. As described by Hodson and Paden (1983, p.4), the phonologic approach "takes advantage of the systematic nature of speech deviations." Since phonology is defined as both the speech sounds and a rule system to govern the use of the sounds, students with articulation disorders are evaluated to determine the defective sounds and the rule system that they use to produce the sounds. Research has demonstrated that the rules governing disordered articulation parallel those rules found in use by younger children. It appears that all speech, normal or disordered, has its own structure and rule system. Knowledge and understanding of this fact has led to the implementation of the phonologic approach to articulation therapy.

This discussion by no means has included all the theories, approaches, and treatment programs used in articulation therapy. Many programs are modifications of those programs presented here. Frequently incorporated in any number of programs is a behavior modification approach that is not exclusive to articulation therapy. The type of program selected for treatment will depend in a large part on the philosophy and training of the speech–language pathologist. But as stated earlier, the major goal of therapy remains the same no matter what approach is chosen.

THE ROLE OF THE CLASSROOM TEACHER

A few decades ago, a number of speech improvement and language development programs in the classroom were conducted to determine whether this approach was truly beneficial. *Without exception, results of the research indicated both the need for and the effectiveness of such programs* (Byrne, 1962; Jones, 1958; Wilson, 1954; Work, 1968). These programs basically were designed to offer all children the opportunity to improve oral language, to eliminate many minor speech problems, and to prevent the development of more serious ones. They were not designed, however, to provide a speech therapy program. There are many programs for both the younger child and the adolescent available today that are readily incorporated into daily classroom activities. The resourceful teacher will find these programs to be a successful addition to the basic curriculum.

Teaming with the Speech–Language Pathologist

The classroom teacher has the opportunity to incorporate speech and language skills into classroom activities and subject matter on a daily basis. Since articulation defects account for a large number of speech and language problems, the preseɪ.ᴛa-tion of listening activities can build awareness of sounds so that the children can learn to identify specific sounds. Learning to listen and learning about listening can benefit children with articulation disorders and at the same time improve the auditory discrimination skills of all children.

The classroom teacher can help the speech–language pathologist by following up the therapy lessons in the classroom. When the speech–language pathologist suggests that the child is ready for some supportive activities in the classroom, the teacher can encourage the child to use the correct sound in reading and speaking. This not only provides carry-over use of the sound in specific situations, but it also assists the child to integrate the newly learned sound into a total speech pattern.

Perhaps the teacher's greatest contribution to the speech–language program is a positive attitude. If the classroom teacher believes in and is enthusiastic about the program, the children will likely share the enthusiasm. Accepting the children and their articulation disorders with understanding is a basic key to helping children improve speech. The ideal classroom climate holds no threat or penalty to the child who cannot measure up orally. The child with an articulation deficit will thrive in a warm, supportive classroom climate.

Techniques for Teaming and Teaching

Many teachers are concerned about how best to help children with speech defects. A major consideration is the classroom environment and the attitude others show toward the student with an articulation problem. Part of the warm, supportive classroom climate is built on helping all the students develop a positive, wholesome attitude about the speech therapy program. This can be accomplished by holding a short class discussion on speech therapy, allowing the students to exchange ideas and ask questions. To enhance this activity, the speech–language pathologist could be invited to speak to the class about the program and to answer questions. As the students progress through therapy, they can be encouraged to prepare and present a report about their lessons to the class. A buddy system can be established whereby a classmate meets with the speech student regularly to assist in practice sessions and to provide information about materials and assignments missed while the student attends therapy sessions.

For younger children, understanding that all development, including speech, is sequential and built on a hierarchy of learning is essential. To demand performance beyond the student's developmental stage can be detrimental. It is important, therefore, to meet with the speech–language pathologist on a regular basis to determine individual skill level and progress of the student in therapy. These meetings may be held informally at the beginning or end of the school day or they may be planned on a more formal basis, as with an individual educational plan (IEP) meeting. In either case, the classroom teacher and the speech–language pathologist are encouraged to seek a meeting whenever it is determined to be necessary or potentially beneficial.

For the older student, meeting on a regular basis offers opportunities to determine which classroom or curriculum activities can best be incorporated in the speech therapy plan. Speech–language pathologists are not expected to teach course content, but by being aware of and using course materials in the therapy session, correct sound production can be reinforced and transferred to regular classroom activities. When the classroom teacher is aware of the student's progress in speech and encourages correct use of the sounds, the student may be less hesitant to participate orally in class.

As students progress through the various stages of therapy, many old behaviors must be unlearned before new ones can be learned. The teacher can reinforce students' current level of proficiency and encourage the next developmental step by keeping the following in mind: (1) allow students to express themselves in their own way; (2) take time to listen and to try to understand what is being said; (3) avoid filling in the words when students are searching for what to say; (4) offer a variety of opportunities for students to talk and to respond to others; (5) serve as a model of good speech by rephrasing students' statements so that the correct sound is presented; and (6) allow the students to be active participants in communication experiences.

SUMMARY

In this chapter, we have examined normal articulation development and factors related to this development. We have defined articulation disorders and considered a variety of causes linked to the disorders. A brief history of treatment programs, their theories and applications, has been presented. The role of prevention, speech improvement programs, and the classroom teacher has been discussed. Hopefully, the suggestions offered to the classroom teacher assisting the speech-disordered student will be useful.

If speech and language skills are emphasized in many learning activities, then speech improvement and language development become an integral part of the student's overall development and enhance efforts for good sound production. All students have basic needs: need for understanding, for acceptance, for growth. The ability to communicate effectively nurtures these needs. By encouraging students to overcome their articulation disorders, teachers will assist in developing an understanding of and appreciation for language and communication.

GLOSSARY

ADDITIONS. In speech, unnecessary or inappropriate sounds that are inserted in a word or in between words, but are not the result of a dialect.

ARTICULATION. The process of forming meaningful oral symbols by the manipulation of the articulators.

ARTICULATORS. The organs of the mouth or throat that help to produce speech: the tongue, lips, lower jaw, teeth, soft palate, and larynx.

AUTISM. A psychological state characterized in degree by daydreaming, preoccupation with fantasy life, retreat from social experiences, and mutism.

CEREBRAL PALSY. Any of several disorders of the central nervous system characterized by spastic paralysis, defective motor ability, and articulation disorders.

CLEFT PALATE. A congenital cleft of the roof of the mouth, which may include the soft palate, the hard palate, or both.

DISTORTIONS. In speech, an approximation of a correct sound that is different enough to be noticeable.

FUNCTIONAL. Referring to speech sound production that is not caused by physical condition and may be due to faulty learning or faulty listening.

LINGUISTIC. Pertaining to the intellectual aspects of language; signifying the ideational background of speech.

LISPING. Defective utterance of sibilant sounds /s/, /z/, /sh/, /zh/; usually refers to defective /s/ and /z/.

OMISSIONS. In speech, a dropping or leaving out of a sound in a word.

PHONEME. The smallest differences in a language that serve to differentiate meanings within the language, for example, /b/, /d/, /k/.

PHONETICS. The science of speech sounds and their production.

PHONOLOGY. The sound structure of language and the rules that govern the structure.

SPEECH. The audible motor production of sounds and sound patterns, including voice quality and rhythm.

SUBSTITUTIONS. In speech, the use of an incorrect sound or a different sound for the one intended for use.

QUESTIONS FOR DISCUSSION

1. How may a classroom teacher determine whether a student might have an articulation disorder?
2. When should a referral for an articulation disorder be made to the speech–language pathologist?
3. What other factors not identified in this chapter would be important to the development of an effective speech improvement, language development program?
4. What are some effective methods to explain the speech–language therapy program to a kindergarten class? a fifth grade class? a senior high class?
5. What principles should guide the teacher in assisting the student with an articulation disorder?
6. How can the teacher identify resources, such as speech improvement programs, to be used in the elementary classroom?
7. Where can a high school teacher locate resources to assist the student with an articulation disorder?
8. What factors contribute to a good working relationship between the teacher and the speech–language pathologist?
9. What regular classroom activities would be effective for incorporating practice material from speech therapy?
10. How may the speech–language pathologist serve as a consultant to the classroom teacher? How may the classroom teacher serve as a consultant to the speech–language pathologist?

REFERENCES

Atkinson M, & Canter G (1979). Variables influencing phonemic discrimination performance in normal and learning disabled children. *Journal of Speech and Hearing Disorders, 44,* 543–556

Backus O, & Beasley J (1951). *Speech therapy with children.* Boston: Houghton Mifflin Company

Berry M, & Eisenson J (1956). *Speech disorders: Principles and practices of therapy.* New York: Appleton-Century-Crofts, Inc.

Byrne M (1962). *Development and evaluation of a speech improvement program for kindergarten and first grade children.* Lawrence, KS: Speech and Hearing Clinic, University of Kansas

Hodson B, & Paden E (1983). *Targeting intelligible speech.* San Diego: College Hill Press

Ingram D (1976). *Phonological disability in children.* New York: Elsevier

Jakobson R, Fant G, & Halle M (1951). *Preliminaries to speech analysis: The distinctive features and their correlates.* Cambridge, MA: M.I.T. Press

Jones R (1958). *For speech sake.* San Francisco: Fearon Publishers

Liberman I, Shankweiler D, Camp L, Heifetz B, & Werfelman J (1977). Steps toward literacy. A report of reading prepared for the *Working Group on Learning Failure and Unused Learning Potential* for the President's Commission on Mental Health, Washington, D.C.

Panagos J (1974). Persistence of the open syllable reinterpreted as a symptom of language disorder. *Journal of Speech and Hearing Disorders, 1,* 23–31

Phillips P (1975). *Speech and hearing problems in the classroom.* Lincoln, NE: Cliffs Notes, Inc

Sander E (1972). When are speech sounds learned? *Journal of Speech and Hearing Disorders, 37,* 55–62

Scripture M, & Jackson E (1927). *A manual of exercises for the correction of speech disorders.* Philadelphia, PA: F.A. Davis Co.

Shriner T, Holloway M, & Daniloff R (1969). The relationship between articulatory deficits and syntax in speech of defective children. *Journal of Speech and Hearing Research, 12,* 319–325

Sommers R, Cockerville C, Paul C, Bowser D, Fichter G, Fenton A, & Copetas F (1961). Effects of speech therapy and speech improvement upon articulation and reading. *Journal of Speech and Hearing Disorders, 26,* 27–38

Sommers R, & Kane A (1974). Nature and remediation of functional articulation disorders. In S. Dickson (Ed.), *Communication disorders: Remedial principles and practices.* Glenview, IL: Scott Foresman & Co.

Stark J, & Wallach G (1980). The path to a concept of language learning disabilities. *Topics in Language Disorders, 1,* 1–14

Stinchfield-Hawk S, & Young E (1938). *Children with delayed or defective speech.* Stanford, CA: Stanford University Press

Templin M (1957). *Certain language skills in children.* Minneapolis, MN: University of Minnesota Press

Van Riper C (1939). *Speech correction: Principles and methods.* (1st ed.) Englewood Cliffs, NJ: Prentice-Hall, Inc.

Van Riper C (1972). *Speech correction: Principles and methods.* (5th ed.) Englewood Cliffs, NJ: Prentice-Hall, Inc.

Whitacre J, Luper H, & Pollio H (1970). General language deficits in children with articulation problems. *Language and Speech, 13,* 231–239

Wilson B (1954). The development and evaluation of a speech improvement program for kindergarten children. *Journal of Speech and Hearing Disorders, 19,* 4–13

Work R (1968). The development and evaluation of a speech improvement program in grades one and two. Unpublished master's thesis, University of Florida, Gainesville, FL

── 13 ───────────────────────────

Hearing Impairment in Children: Causation, Assessment, and Treatment

Allan O. Diefendorf
Ralph G. Leverett

EDITOR'S INTRODUCTION

Drs. Diefendorf and Leverett are respected professionals who are familiar with the aural problems and habilitation of elementary- and adolescent-age children. Their two chapters address these matters. Both authors have had significant interactions with teachers and are cognizant of their needs for information on aural disorders in childhood.

As is pointed out in Chapter 7, there is a marked deficiency in teachers' understanding of hearing loss and its implications. The following chapters should help to eliminate this deficiency.

Identifying the etiology of oral communication problems is desirable prior to establishing suitable treatment plans, particularly if an auditory disorder and hearing impairment is suspected. While the deficits imposed by impaired hearing have implications for the development of social, academic, and vocational skills, the most devastating effect of hearing impairment is the impact on verbal communication.

Concern about the possibility of hearing impairment is dependent on those individuals whom children revolve around: parents, educators, and physicians. If this triad of individuals is aware of hearing impairment in children, and educational problems that may ensue, amelioration of subsequent aural/oral communication problems can be initiated early.

This chapter is intended specifically for educators, who at different times may be pivotal in this triad. Young children with severe to profound congenital hearing impairments usually are identified by parents and/or physicians. However, when there is a lesser degree of hearing loss, still resulting in disordered speech and

ORAL COMMUNICATION PROBLEMS
IN CHILDREN AND ADOLESCENTS
Copyright © 1988 by Grune & Stratton, Inc.

ISBN 0-8089-1887-7
All rights reserved.

language reception and expression, parents and educators must bear the responsibility of insuring early and proper identification. This requires educators to possess knowledge of certain aspects of hearing impairment. The purpose of this chapter is to assist educators in acquiring knowledge in the areas of causation, assessment, and treatment of hearing impairment in children.

CAUSATION

Prevalence of Hearing Loss

Hearing loss occurs in one of 50–56 infants in the neonatal intensive care nursery (McFarland, Simmons, & Jones, 1980; Schulman-Galambos & Galambos, 1979) and one in 700–2000 infants in the "well" nursery (Northern & Downs, 1974; Stewart, 1979). These reports only represent severe hearing loss, so the actual incidence of all degrees of hearing loss in infants and children would be significantly greater. When children with milder forms of hearing loss are included, the prevalence rate rises sharply and is estimated to involve 15–30 times more children. The well known Pittsburgh study (Eagles, Wishik, & Doerfler, 1967) has reported that about 50 out of every 1000 school children (5 percent) exhibit reduced hearing levels in either one or both ears. In 1970, Berg estimated that there were as many as 950,000 hard-of-hearing children having losses in the 26–55 dB (mild to moderate) hearing loss range, who would require assistance in the classroom. That figure has probably grown significantly over the past 17 years with the mounting evidence pointing out the effects of unilateral (one ear), minimal, and high frequency hearing losses on speech and language development and academic achievement.

According to Northern and Downs (1978) the presence of middle-ear disease among children two years and younger increases the frequency of impairment to 1 in 25. Data from studies on screening for ear disease in school children suggest that the prevalence of ear disease is much greater than that of hearing loss. Based on a survey of 3,197 children between the ages of newborn and five years, Klein (1978) estimated that the occurrence of middle-ear disease ranged between 8 to 25 percent. Jerger (1980) stated that middle-ear effusion (otitis media with fluid), the primary middle-ear disorder causing hearing loss in children, ranges up to 30 percent, and has seldom been less than 15 percent. This prevalence rate implies that there may be 2,500,000 children between the ages of newborn and six years in the United States affected by middle-ear disease. When older children and adolescents are included this number is further increased.

Function and Dysfunction of the Ear

The human ear can be divided into three main portions: the outer ear, the middle ear, and the inner ear (see Fig. 13-1). The brain (brainstem and cortex) is the fourth portion and the final stop for acoustic information but is not traditionally

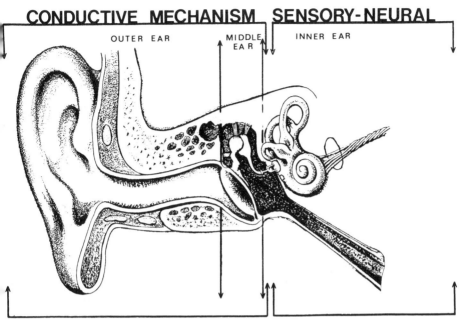

CONDUCTIVE MECHANISM SENSORY-NEURAL

OUTER EAR   MIDDLE   INNER EAR
                      EAR

Fig. 13-1. The human ear divided into three main portions (outer, middle, inner ear).

represented as part of the ear itself. These anatomic divisions are then described as the conductive hearing mechanism, the sensory-neural hearing mechanism (Fig. 13-1), and the central hearing mechanism (see Fig. 13-2).

The conductive hearing mechanism is made up of the external ear (pinna), the eardrum (tympanic membrane), and the middle ear (see Fig. 13-3). This part of the ear is intended anatomically and physiologically to conduct sound vibrations to the sensory-neural mechanism. Any interruption in this function is described as a *conductive hearing loss.* The conductive mechanism is essentially a mechanical system.

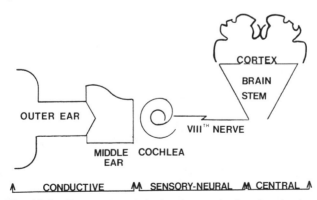

CORTEX

BRAIN STEM

OUTER EAR

VIIITH NERVE

MIDDLE COCHLEA
EAR

CONDUCTIVE   SENSORY-NEURAL CENTRAL

Fig. 13-2. Description of the hearing mechanism (conductive, sensory-neural, central hearing mechanism).

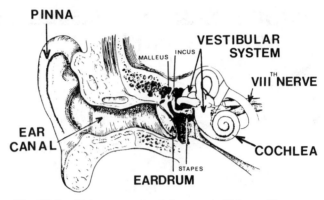

Fig. 13-3. Major structures of the outer, middle, and inner ear.

Sound energy passes through the ear canal and strikes the eardrum (tympanic membrane). The sound waves cause the tympanic membrane to vibrate, in turn creating a mechanical transfer of energy across the middle ear because of the attachment of the tympanic membrane with the three small bones (malleus, incus, stapes) housed within the middle ear. The stapes transfers the mechanical energy to the sensory-neural mechanism. The mechanical action of the middle ear provides a very efficient transfer of energy from the airborne sounds of the ear canal to the fluid medium of the sensory-neural mechanism. The sensory-neural mechanism is made up of the cochlea and the auditory nerve (cranial nerve VIII). Any hearing loss caused by dysfunction of the sensory-neural mechanism is called a *sensory-neural hearing loss.*

The primary function of the sensory-neural mechanism is to conduct sound from the middle ear to the central hearing mechanism that is responsible for the recognition, interpretation, and integration of acoustic information. The sound collected at the middle ear is in the form of mechanical energy. The central nervous system, however, is stimulated by energy in the form of neural (electrical) impulses that are electrochemical in nature. Therefore, in order to transfer sounds from the middle ear to the central hearing mechanism, the sensory-neural mechanism must transform mechanical energy to neurologic (electrical) impulses. This operation is performed in the cochlea. The VIIIth nerve transmits the impulses to the brainstem where they enter the central hearing mechanism. The auditory pathways through the brainstem and the auditory areas in the cortex are referred to as the central hearing mechanism. Damage to this portion of the mechanism may result in a *central hearing loss.* This type of loss causes an inability to recognize, utilize, or understand acoustic information, rather than the loss of sensitivity that is characteristic of conductive or sensory-neural losses. The term peripheral is used in opposition to central; therefore the peripheral hearing mechanism refers to the entire conductive and sensory-neural mechanism.

The audiogram (see Fig. 13-4) is useful for differentiating various types of hearing losses and their severity. Sounds ranging in intensity from 0–110 dB and in

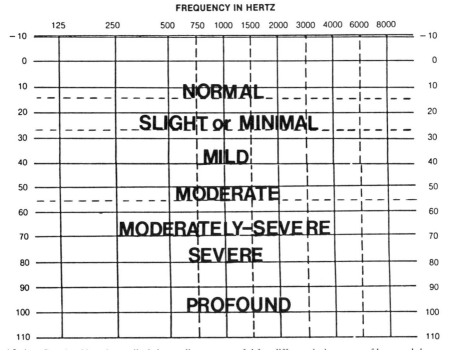

FREQUENCY IN HERTZ

Fig. 13-4. Graph of hearing called the audiogram; useful for differentiating type of loss and degree of loss.

frequency from 125–8000 Hz are presented. The right and left ears are tested separately to determine whether the hearing loss is unilateral or bilateral. The sounds are first presented through the earphones (air conduction) and then through a bone oscillator (bone conduction) attached to the mastoid bone behind the ear (see Fig. 13-5). Administering air conduction and bone conduction tests helps the examiner distinguish between a conductive and a sensory-neural hearing loss. Individuals

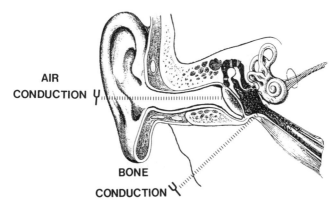

Fig. 13-5. Cross section of ear showing air-conduction (AC) and bone-conduction (BC) pathways.

with a sensory-neural loss have an equal loss of hearing by both tests (threshold levels are equivalent); those with a conductive loss will show a difference, hearing better with the bone oscillator because it allows the sound to bypass the outer and the middle ear where the conductive hearing loss is located.

Major Conductive Disorders in School-Age Children

The Outer Ear

Malformations of the pinna have little effect on hearing, and any such abnormalities are primarily the concern of a plastic surgeon. Surgery to correct the defect is usually considered after age five, but is certainly not considered for every case. Ear canal malformations are sometimes associated with other congenital abnormalities of the tympanic membrane and the middle-ear structures. Although it is sometimes possible to correct an ear canal malformation with surgery, complications such as associated middle-ear malformations often make this type of surgery difficult.

If ear wax (cerumen) collects and hardens in the external auditory canal (impacted cerumen) in sufficient quantities to completely block the flow of sound, a hearing loss will result. This type of loss is temporary with normal hearing returning when the blockage is removed. When the skin of the external auditory meatus becomes inflamed and infected, this condition is referred to as external otitis, a condition that does not normally produce a hearing loss unless the swelling is sufficient to completely close the external auditory canal.

The Tympanic Membrane

Perforations to the tympanic membrane produce a hearing loss that varies greatly depending upon the size and exact location of the perforation. Small, regular perforations tend to heal spontaneously, while larger or irregular perforations are more likely to form scar tissue.

The Middle Ear

In some children, middle-ear pathology (otitis media) may be related to inadequate ventilation of the tympanic cavity due to dysfunction or obstruction of the Eustachian tube. Some causes of Eustachian tube dysfunction include allergy, enlarged tonsils and adenoids, and cleft palate. Negative middle-ear pressure due to inadequate ventilation results in swelling (edema) of the mucosa and secretion of fluid from the lining of the middle ear (mucoperiosteum). At times, instead of the thin, watery fluid (serous otitis media), the fluid (effusion) is a thick, dense, noninfected composition. This is referred to as glue ear (mucoid otitis media).

If an infection invades the middle ear, instead of a clear fluid the middle ear fills with pus. The primary source of these bacteria is through the nose and mouth, although perforation of the tympanic membrane may also allow the infection to enter the middle ear. This infection of the middle ear is known as purulent otitis media or suppurative otitis media, and the condition is often accompanied by pain.

Other Middle Ear Disorders

We have by no means exhausted the list of all possible pathologic conditions of the conductive mechanism. Several others that are important to be aware of will be mentioned briefly.

The cholesteatoma (also called keratoma) is a tissue mass that may occur in any part of the temporal bone but which characteristically occurs in the cavity of the middle ear. The exact reason why these structures form is not really known. The method of formation is apparently related to the shedding of tissue from around the surface of a tympanic membrane perforation. Material being shed is composed primarily of keratin and is a favorable medium for culturing bacteria. As a general rule, cholesteatoma or keratoma develops as a complication of recurrent or long-term middle-ear infection. On rare occasions, however, these tissue masses may occur with no apparent predisposing middle-ear abnormality.

Head trauma can result in a separation of the bones (ossicular chain) in the middle ear or the fracture of a single ossicle. This is known as an ossicular discontinuity. Sudden blows to the head, usually from automobile accidents, are the primary cause of ossicular discontinuities. Long-term middle-ear infections, however, can also cause ossicular discontinuity or decay of tissue or bone (ossicular necrosis).

Major Sensory-Neural Disorders in School-Age Children

It is common clinically to subdivide sensory-neural hearing losses at the cochlea and beyond the cochlea (along the pathway of the VIIIth nerve), depending on the location of the lesion causing the hearing loss. If the hearing loss at the cochlea or beyond the cochlea is caused by damage to the mechanism before birth, the loss is referred to as congenital, as opposed to acquired hearing losses that develop anytime postnatally.

Hereditary Hearing Loss

One of the most common forms of congenital sensory-neural hearing loss is genetically transmitted hearing loss. Hereditary hearing losses can occur as a part of a pattern of symptoms (e.g., blindness, mental impairment), or in isolation where the hearing loss is the only abnormality present.

In most cases the hearing loss associated with genetic abnormalities is present at birth. However, it is recognized that genetic hearing losses can also be progressive; that is, hearing may be near normal at birth, and later in childhood or adolescence hearing becomes progressively poorer.

Nonhereditary Hearing Loss

While 50 percent of the children with congenital hearing loss have a genetic etiology, 50 percent of congenital hearing losses have an unknown etiology. A variety of nonhereditary problems can occur during the prenatal period that may affect the normal development of hearing. Viral infections that may have an effect on the hearing mechanism include rubella (German measles) and cytomegalovirus (CMV).

While rubella is of minimal concern to an adult afflicted with it, this viral infection is a matter of great concern when contracted during pregnancy. Although the danger is greatest during the first three months of pregnancy, injury to the fetus can occur later in pregnancy. CMV is far more common today than prenatal rubella. Since hyperbilirubinemia (Rh incompatibility) is a common manifestation of congenital CMV infection, monitoring the bilirubin level is one way to be alerted to potential hearing loss in newborns who might develop a hearing loss associated with CMV.

Ototoxic poisoning (drugs that are ingested during pregnancy) may affect the hearing mechanism of the fetus, although research in this area is often inconclusive. Damage to the auditory system resulting from maternal ingestion of ototoxic drugs includes middle-ear anomalies, absence of VIIth and VIIIth nerves, and severe damage to the microstructure of the cochlea.

Birth trauma with anoxia (a lack of sufficient oxygen during the birth process) is a cause of central nervous system damage and sometimes results in sensory-neural hearing loss. Anoxia is often associated with premature delivery, head trauma to the infant during delivery, or insufficient oxygen to the fetus due to the umbilical cord being twisted around the neck.

The majority of hearing-impaired individuals incur their hearing loss postnatally, hence their hearing loss is said to be adventitious. The following list of disorders can result in hearing loss at any time from early childhood to late adolescence and on into adult life.

Systemic disorders.   All of those diseases, conditions, and pathologies that affect the general metabolic system and/or chemical homeostasis have a potential for resulting in hearing impairment. Within this group, for example, are such diverse problems as thyroid disease, kidney disease, and diabetes.

Acquired disease.   Viral, bacterial, and protozoal infections can result in damage to the sensory-neural mechanism. These hearing losses can affect one or both ears and can vary in degree from mild hearing loss to a total loss of hearing.

Degenerative disorders.   Some genetically based hearing disorders that are not present at birth appear early in life. These hearing losses come under the general headings of early-onset recessive deafness and early-onset dominant deafness. There is some controversy over the term "early" because it is not really known at what age the hearing loss develops.

Ototoxicity.   Certain medications may permanently injure or destroy the microstructure of the cochlea, thus creating a sensory hearing impairment. Different ototoxic drugs may include kanamycin, neomycin, vancomycin, and streptomycin. Aspirin in prolonged use is also known to be ototoxic, but its effects are often at least partially reversible when the drug is withdrawn. Children (as well as adults) who have impaired kidney (renal) function are particularly susceptible to all ototoxic drugs, because the drug is allowed to remain in the individual system long after it should have been excreted by normal kidney function.

Noise trauma. A sound of sufficient intensity and duration can cause injury to the ear producing temporary or permanent hearing loss. The extent of noise-induced hearing loss in children is difficult to determine. However, a number of devices used by children produce sound intensity levels capable of producing permanent injury to the ear. A list of those devices would include stereo headphones, video arcade games, firecrackers, toy firearms, and gasoline powered engines. Because individual susceptibility to hearing loss from noise exposure exists, caution must be exercised in exposing young ears to a loud sound.

Disorders of the Central Auditory Mechanism

The symptoms of a central hearing disorder are often vague and difficult to define. The correlation of symptoms with specific anatomic damage is often impossible. Sometimes the damage is clearly localized, like a tumor in the brain or brainstem; at other times the damage is diffused, as in arteriosclerosis. A degenerative disease such as multiple sclerosis can also account for central hearing disorders. Unlike a peripheral disorder, patients with a central hearing loss will not normally have the loss of hearing sensitivity that is usually associated with hearing disorders. However, central hearing disorders manifest themselves as problems in interpretation, integration, and/or appropriate utilization of the acoustic information.

Hearing Loss Characteristics

Important characteristics of hearing as they relate to management include: (1) degree of hearing loss, (2) type of hearing loss, (3) time of onset, and (4) auditory perception.

Degree of Loss

In 1975, the Conference of Executives of American Schools for the Deaf adopted the following definitions:

Hearing impairment. A generic term indicating a hearing disability which may range in severity from mild to profound: it includes the subsets of deaf and hard of hearing.

Deaf person. A deaf person is one whose hearing disability precludes successful processing of linguistic information through audition, with or without a hearing aid.

Hard-of-hearing person. A hard-of-hearing person is one who, generally with the use of a hearing aid, has residual hearing sufficient to enable successful processing of linguistic information through audition.

It is not possible to draw firm boundaries between the deaf and the hard of hearing on the basis of severity of loss shown on an audiogram. The following classification system, however, based on the average of pure tone hearing threshold levels of 500, 1000, and 2000 Hz, is a general guide to degree of severity of hearing losses (refer to Fig. 13-4):

zero – 15 dB	normal
16 – 25 dB	slight or minimal hearing loss
26 – 40 dB	mild hearing loss
41 – 55 dB	moderate hearing loss
56 – 70 dB	moderately severe hearing loss
71 – 90 dB	severe hearing loss
> 90 dB	profound hearing loss

Knauf (1978) made the following observation about the degree of loss:

> The hearing threshold level is perhaps the primary variable for estimating the impact of a child's hearing impairment and it frequently is the first measure available. It is not surprising then that judgements and classifications of the hearing impaired are sometimes based only on this criterion. While classifications based on hearing level are valuable in estimating the impact of a certain hearing level on an average child and in the early counseling of parents, there are many exceptions. Some unusual children with profound losses of 90 dB perform better in language and academic skills compared to other children with average intelligence and moderately-severe [sic] losses of 70 dB. Similar individual variations will be found along the entire continuum of hearing levels. (p 550)

Type of Loss

The type of loss may be conductive (with damage in the outer and middle ears), sensory-neural (with impairment in the inner ear or nerve of hearing), or mixed (a combination of both conductive and sensory-neural). A less common type of hearing loss is a central hearing disorder (which arises from the central nervous system or brain and brainstem).

Conductive hearing loss is of more widespread concern because the incidence is greater, and these losses may be responsible for articulation disorders, voice problems, language and learning disorders, as well as behavior problems. Sensory-neural hearing losses are more distressing because of the life-long impact the hearing loss may have on communication, academic, vocational, and psychological development. Hearing loss is not usually associated with central hearing loss; however, the processing of speech and language may be impaired in varying degrees. Thus, teachers must be astute observers of communication skills (language, articulation, voice) and behavior (shy, withdrawn, "doesn't pay attention") in order to identify early the possible existence of a hearing loss or ear disorder.

Time of Onset

The degree of handicap produced by hearing loss depends to a considerable extent on its time of onset. Hearing impairment may be divided into three catagories (prelingual, postlingual, deafened), depending on the age at which the loss occurs. Prelingual deafness refers to impairment that is present at birth or shortly thereafter. The longer a person has normal hearing during the crucial language development years up to age five, the less chance there is that language development will be delayed. Postlingual deafness means that the loss occurs after about age five and is generally less serious. Even though language may be less affected, speech and education may be affected substantially. Deafened persons are those who lose hearing after their schooling is completed, that is, in their late teen years or thereafter. Normal speech, language, and education are possible for those individuals, but difficulty in verbal communication and other social, emotional, and vocational problems will likely occur (Table 13-1).

Auditory Perception

Auditory perception is another important dimension of hearing loss. The auditory perception (maximum development of residual hearing for listening skill development) of the hard-of-hearing individual typically is better than for a deaf person. The deaf are generally considered unable to comprehend conversational speech in most situations, whereas the hard of hearing can use their residual hearing to some extent for speech recognition and language comprehension. A description of auditory perception must include the segmental aspects of speech and the suprasegmental aspects (rhythm, intonation, stress, and pause) of speech when determining the effects of hearing loss on the individual's auditory perception.

ASSESSMENT

Screening

The purpose of screening is to identify as early as possible those individuals having a defined disorder who would not have been identified otherwise (Silverman, Lane, & Calvert, 1978). Screening can be viewed as the general process by which groups of people are separated into those who manifest some defined trait, or those who do not. The outcome of screening is incomplete if it is not followed up with the administration of appropriate treatment at a time when it will either remedy the disorder or impede its rate of development.

Despite the compelling need for early identification, the vast majority of screening programs occur at the school-age level. This is unfortunate, particularly when considering the critical importance of the first two years for the development of speech and language. Once newborns leave the hospital it is not until age five, at the kindergarten level, that these children can be tested at one common location.

Newborns

Over the past decade, programs and procedures for screening the hearing of newborns have been developed, modified, and improved. Clearly, the screening for

Table 13-1

Handicapping Effects of Hearing Loss

Average Hearing 500–2,000 (ANSI)	Description	Possible Condition	What Can be Heard Without Amplification	Handicapping Effects (If Not Treated in 1st Year of Life)	Probable Needs
0–15 dB	Normal range	Conductive hearing losses	All speech sounds	None	None
15–25 dB	Slight hearing loss	Conductive hearing losses, some sensorineural hearing losses	Vowel sounds heard clearly; may miss unvoiced consonant sounds	Mild auditory dysfunction in language learning	Consideration of need for hearing aid; speech reading, auditory training, speech therapy, preferential seating
25–40 dB	Mild hearing loss	Conductive or sensorineural hearing loss	Only some of speech sounds, the louder voiced sounds	Auditory learning dysfunction, mild language retardation, mild speech problems, inattention	Hearing aid, speech reading, auditory training, speech therapy
40–65 dB	Moderate hearing loss	Conductive hearing loss from chronic middle-ear disorders; sensorineural hearing losses	Almost no speech sounds at normal conversational level	Speech problems, language retardation, learning dysfunction, inattention	All of the above, plus consideration of special classroom situation
69–95 dB	Severe hearing loss	Sensorineural or mixed losses due to a combination of middle-ear disease and sensorineural involvement	No speech sounds of normal conversations	Severe speech problems, language retardation, learning dysfunction, inattention	All of the above; probable assignment to special classes
95 dB+	Profound hearing loss	Sensorineural or mixed losses due to a combination of middle-ear disease and sensorineural involvement	No speech or other sounds	Severe speech problems, language retardation, learning dysfunction, inattention	All of the above; probable assignment to special classes

Source: Reprinted from Northern, JL., & Lemme M (1986). Hearing and auditory disorders. In GH Shames & EH Wiig (Eds), *Human communication disorders* (p 432). Columbus, OH: Charles E. Merrill. With permission.

any disorder is a task that should be accomplished rapidly, accurately, economically, and with little energy for resources misspent pursuing the so-called normals. No diagnostic screening device fulfills these criteria completely. However, the high-risk register, the crib-o-gram, and the auditory brainstem response (see Table 13-2) are instruments that have been used in the newborn nursery so that hearing loss in neonates can be identified early. Further, when developmental milestones for hearing are targeted and recognized by pediatricians, parents, and early educators particularly during the first two years of life, follow-up needs of infants suspected of hearing loss can be met more easily.

Preschool Children

Screening the preschool child also has several distinct advantages. As children get older, they become easier to test. Moreover, children with delayed hereditary

Table 13-2
Three Different Screening Devices Utilized in the Newborn Nursery

Diagnostic Screening Device	Description of Procedure	Effectiveness
High-risk registry	The use of a seven-item questionnaire for determining a subgroup at-risk for hearing loss. (1) Familial deafness, (2) rubella during pregnancy, (3) birth weight < 1500 grams, (4) congenital malformations (ear, nose, throat), (5) hyperbilirubinemia, (6) severe neonatal infections, and (7) apgar score 4–7	60–75% of children with severe hearing losses should be identified
Crib-o-gram	Automated device that measures an infant's startle response. A graphic recorder automatically records infant motor activity prior to, during, and immediately following presentation of auditory test stimuli.	Assesses 91% of neonatal intensive care unit (NICU) infants; false–positive rate is approximately 15% (major limitation: 93 dB screening intensity).
Auditory brainstem response (ABR)	Brief latency multiphasic electrophysiologic response that is considered to reflect the electrical activity of the auditory nerve and successive brainstem structures. Recorded from scalp electrodes and summed by computer.	Extremely sensitive procedure for detecting hearing loss *except* when there may be disorders of neurologic development, maturation, or function. In these cases false–positives are significantly increased.

hearing loss, who give no evidence of hearing loss at birth by history or objective screening, may be recognized early. Finally, hearing-impaired children who move into a community would have a chance to be identified.

School-Age Children

The purposes of a school hearing conservation program are to reduce to the absolute minimum the number of children with permanently impaired hearing and to provide for the special education needs of children whose hearing cannot be restored to normal through medical or surgical treatment. Because the discovery of children with hearing losses is prerequisite to providing for their needs, hearing screening is at the heart of hearing conservation. It is usually true that in the first two or three years of a hearing conservation program, testing may lead to the classification of as many as 10 percent of the school population as having "medically significant" hearing losses, whereas after the program has been in effect for a few years, this number may be reduced to a level of 3–5 percent. In any school system, the greatest number of medically significant hearing losses will be discovered in the primary grades, for the reason that very young children have a higher incidence of upper respiratory infections, tonsil and adenoid problems, Eustachian tube dysfunction and allergy problems. Because these conditions usually respond to proper medical treatment, it is important that they be discovered as soon as they become evident. In its early years, therefore, a hearing conservation program should concentrate on the primary grades. The discovery and treatment of conditions producing hearing loss will then reduce the number of hearing losses in the higher elementary grades and in junior and senior high school.

The basic instrument needed for hearing screening is the portable screening audiometer. Portable audiometers are manufactured by numerous special instrument companies and are relatively inexpensive. They must be recalibrated at regular intervals depending on usage. The screening levels recommended by the American Speech, Language, and Hearing Association are 20 dB at 1000, 2000, and 4000 Hz. If the 20 dB tone is not heard at 4000 Hz, a 25 dB screening tone can be used. Hearing screening tests should be conducted by someone who has had appropriate training and should be done in a quiet room away from street noises, foot traffic, visual distractions, and other disturbances, which may result in an inaccurate or unreliable hearing test.

Acoustic immittance is not a test of hearing, per se, but a technique used to evaluate the function of the auditory system (specifically the middle ear). Various ear disorders can be identified with the acoustic immittance test battery, which includes tympanometry (measurement of eardrum mobility) and middle-ear muscles reflex evaluation.

The literature is now replete with studies showing why screening for middle-ear disorders in school children is needed. The most notable finding is unanimous documentation that pure tone screening tests are not sensitive to middle-ear disorders. Moreover, these studies have shown that immittance measures increase the overall accuracy of a screening program, reduce the number of children who must be retested prior to referral, and increase the likelihood that all children who are referred for medical examination have valid otologic problems. Although research data support the use of immittance screening to detect middle-ear disorders in school children, the extreme sensitivity of the test has caused high false–positive (test failed with normal ear) rates for a large number of programs. Despite this factor, immittance screening should be a part of any comprehensive school hearing conservation program.

Evaluation

The major goal of hearing assessment is to identify the type and the degree of hearing loss. Age-appropriate testing techniques must be employed to insure accurate assessment of the hearing mechanism (see Table 13-3). After the appropriate testing strategy has been decided upon, the basic hearing evaluation is similar across different age groups.

The basic hearing evaluation includes pure tone air and bone conduction tests, as well as speech tests. Air conduction tests refer to the measurement of hearing

Table 13-3
Age-Appropriate Test Techniques

	Test Technique	Appropriate Age	Response Task
Audiometry	Visual reinforcement audiometry (VRA)	6–24 months (developmentally)	45 or 90° Head-turn (localization)
	Tangible reinforcement operant-conditioning audiometry (TROCA)	18–30 months	Bar-press
	Conditioned play audiometry	30 months–4 years	Stacking blocks, pegs-in-the-board, simple puzzles, rings on a tower
	Conditioned hand-raising/finger-raising response	>4–5 years	Same as technique
Speech reception	Speech reception threshold (SRT)	2–3 years	Simple commands, identify body parts, point to common toys
	Speech reception threshold (SRT)	4–6 years	Reception of selected words (children's spondee list)
	Speech reception threshold	>6 years	Children's spondee list

thresholds with signals heard through earphones or sound field speakers, and all parts of the hearing mechanism are assessed.

Bone conduction assessment determines the lowest level of response for the test frequencies 250 through 4000 Hz. On the basis of air conduction and bone conduction comparisons, the type of hearing loss (conductive, sensory-neural, mixed) is identified (see Fig. 13-6). When air conduction and bone conduction thresholds are equal, a sensory-neural hearing loss is indicated; when bone conduction is normal, with air conduction responses depressed on the audiogram, a conductive hearing loss is indicated. If air conduction and bone conduction are depressed, but a difference exists between the two tests, a mixed hearing loss is indicated.

Each audiologic evaluation includes some assessment of hearing using speech as the stimulus. The audiologist attempts to measure two speech quantities: speech reception thresholds (SRT) and speech recognition. The SRT is established as the lowest (softest) level in dB at which individuals can correctly repeat two-syllable words. Some indication of degree of hearing loss is reflected in the SRT. Speech recognition ability is the percentage of syllables, monosyllabic words, or sentences the patient can correctly identify when the stimuli are presented at a comfortable listening level under ideal (quiet) conditions. Slightly depressed speech recognition scores should serve as an immediate sign to classroom teachers that actual performance will be even poorer because of the noise levels and reverberant (echo) conditions of most classrooms.

The immittance test battery is an important part of every audiometric evaluation. Although each test of the immittance measurement battery provides some information about the functional integrity of the auditory system, the results are most meaningful when relationships among tests are considered in reference to the pure tone and speech audiometric evaluation.

TREATMENT

Medical Management

Once a hearing loss has been detected or evaluated by an audiologist, the individual should be referred for medical evaluation by a physician trained to treat disorders of the ears, nose, and throat (an otolaryngologist). Some hearing losses can be remedied by medical intervention involving drugs and surgery, but many cannot.

Conductive Hearing Loss

Conductive hearing losses can be eliminated or substantially improved by medical treatment. Conditions that involve blockage of the outer ear, such as excessive earwax, foreign bodies, or external otitis, can be remedied by their removal. The most common source of conductive hearing loss is otitis media, for which medical

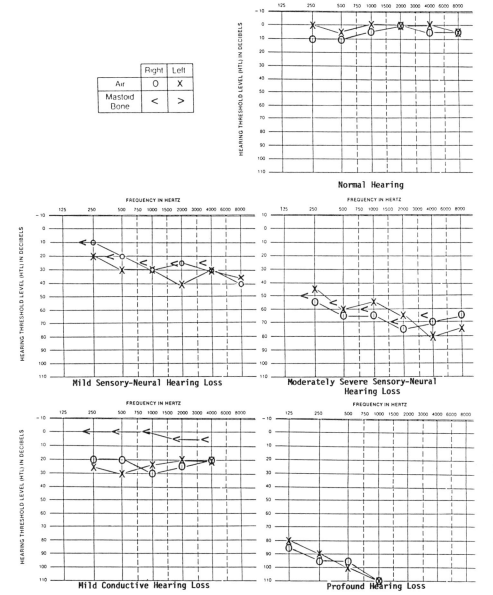

Fig. 13-6. Audiograms showing normal hearing and various degrees of hearing loss.

treatment consisting of antibiotics, decongestants, and analgesics can be used to reduce swelling and congestion about the Eustachian tube and provide better drainage of the middle ear via that route.

In the early stages of otitis media antibiotic medication may be prescribed to prevent bacterial growth. In the latter stages, in addition to prescribing antibiotics, the otolaryngologist may make an incision in the tympanic membrane (myringotomy). A myringotomy can give an immediate relief of pain, and the drainage initiates recovery from the disease. Ventilating tubes may be fitted through the eardrum if the otitis media is chronic.

There are several operations that can be used for chronic otitis media. These vary from an operation designed to repair a perforation of the tympanic membrane (myringoplasty), to hollowing out the mastoid process (tympanomastoidectomy). Mastoid surgery is generally reserved for those patients with cholesteatoma or keratoma and mastoid infections.

Sensory-Neural Hearing Loss

When the onset of sensory-neural hearing loss is sudden, a medical referral for examination and possible treatment is absolutely essential. In some cases of sensory-neural hearing loss (e.g., ototoxicity, metabolic disorders), medical intervention may alleviate the hearing loss. However, most hearing losses of sensory-neural origin are not remedied by medical intervention. In cases of confirmed sensory-neural hearing loss of a permanent nature, audiologic rehabilitation is recommended.

Audiologic Management

Audiologic management differs considerably between congenitally or prelingually hearing-impaired children and hearing-impaired adults with established communication skills. Treatment plans are broadly divided into two categories: habilitation and rehabilitation. The term rehabilitation is intended to describe programs for individuals whose hearing loss has been acquired after communication skills (speech and language) have been well established. Habilitation describes programs for children with hearing loss present at birth or acquired before communication skills are developed.

Treatment plans for sensory-neural hearing loss include medical intervention, speech and language therapy emphasizing both receptive and expressive language, special services to meet educational, social, vocational, and psychologic needs, and hearing aid amplification. According to Ross (1975), "the early, appropriate, and supervised use of hearing aid amplification is the single most effective rehabilitation tool we have" (p 131) to assist the hearing impaired child. It is true that some patients with hearing loss do not need or cannot use a hearing aid. An audiologist should nevertheless examine this possibility for all patients as part of the total habilitation/rehabilitation program.

Amplification

Hearing aids (Fig. 13-7) are usually described in terms of how sounds are amplified (electroacoustic properties). Specifically, each of the following variables merits careful consideration: the amount of increased loudness (gain) needed across frequency to assure audibility of the full sound range (acoustic spectrum) of speech; maximum loudness (maximum power output) to prevent either temporary or permanent threshold shifts; and the type of hearing aid.

Body-Type Hearing Aids

Body-type hearing aids contain the microphone, amplifier, tone and power controls, and battery in a case that may be clipped to the wearer's clothing or worn in a pocket or a special harness. With the rapidly changing technology in hearing aid amplification, there appears to be only one major advantage of the body-type hearing aids: the controls are easy to adjust because they are relatively large—more of a convenience for geriatric hearing aid users as opposed to children or adolescents.

Behind-the-Ear Hearing Aids

Hearing aids worn behind-the-ear (BTE) are now appropriate for almost all types and degrees of hearing loss. Problems of clothing noise are eliminated with BTE aids, as are difficulties with the cords, because the receiver is built into the

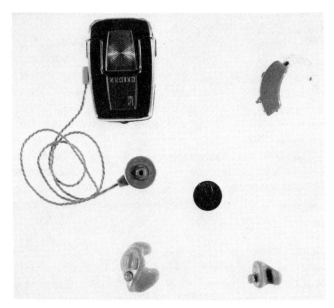

Fig. 13-7. Four different styles of hearing aids. (Clockwise from top right: body-type; behind-the-ear (BTE); in-the-ear (ITE); canal aid.)

same case that houses the microphone and amplifier. They allow somewhat for localization of sound, especially when a separate instrument is worn on each ear (binaural). The decreased size of the instrument makes adjustments of controls and insertion of batteries somewhat more difficult, especially for patients who are very young or physically handicapped.

In-the-Ear Hearing Aids

The most recently introduced hearing aid is the in-the-ear (ITE) type. The entire hearing aid is built within the plastic shell of an earmold. With improved technology the gain, output, and frequency–response characteristics of ITE aids have been vastly improved, but are still restricted in terms of the degree and configuration of hearing loss for which they will be useful. Children with losses greater than moderately severe are not considered for ITE aids.

The newest type of hearing aid to have a major impact is the canal aid, which fits primarily in the external auditory canal with only slight protrusion into the pinna. This design takes advantage of the natural acoustic properties of the pinna, which are largely ignored by the other instrument styles. One obvious advantage to the canal aid is cosmetic appeal; it is almost entirely concealed.

Any of the hearing aids just described can be worn in one ear or in both ears, barring anatomic abnormalities or restrictive hearing loss. Many audiologists have been convinced, either through their research or through comments by their patients, that speech is clearer, louder, easier to understand, and less contaminated by background noise when two hearing aids are worn.

Auditory Trainers

Hearing aids and auditory trainers operate on the same electronic principles and both are used in the habilitation/rehabilitation of the hearing-impaired patient. Although auditory trainers are closely related to hearing aids, and are sometimes referred to as nonwearable hearing aids, there are several important distinctions between them. Most often auditory trainers serve not as a hearing device in everyday listening, but rather as a training device to be used in the classroom. Their major advantage for use as a training device is in providing a clear signal to the student relatively free from any background noise. There are four basic types of auditory trainers: portable desk models, hard-wire units, induction loop units, and FM radio frequency units.

Desk trainers. Desk trainers are built in a small metal case, which is generally positioned on the student's desk. Flexible cords lead from the enclosure to hearing aid receivers or to large earphones in cushions. The desk model has a gain control, and some also have frequency–response and output controls that can be adjusted by the teacher or student. The device is portable, so the child can carry the auditory trainer around the classroom if necessary.

Hard-wire units. In the hard-wire units the teacher speaks into a microphone. The amplified signal is led to any number of units at the children's desks. The child typically has an individual volume control, although in some units there is only a master volume control, which is generally adjusted by the teacher. Connected to the child's amplifier are the same type of cords with receiver or earphones that are used in the desk type units.

Induction loop system. The induction loop system has been popular in classrooms for the hearing-impaired. This system involves a wire loop around the room, attached to the wall, under the outer wall, under the outer edge of a carpet, or even permanently mounted under a tile floor. A heavy current, or electromagnetic energy runs through the wire loop resulting in a magnetic field around the loop, which fills the room if it is not too large. The child wears a personal hearing aid set to the telephone position for input. The telephone coil in the hearing aid will pick up the audio signal by transformer action, amplify it, and present it to the ear as if it were picked up by the microphone. The loop system is flexible inasmuch as the child can move anywhere within the room and still pick up the signal.

FM frequency units. The most recent development in auditory training systems is the FM radio frequency type of unit. These wireless units were introduced several years ago and are now widely used. The FM system consists of a teacher's microphone, which broadcasts by FM directly to the children's wearable units on a frequency-modulated radio carrier wave. There are no wires around the classroom nor installation of any sort.

Following the placement of amplification, a therapy program aimed at improving the child's language skills and communication system must be initiated. The exceptional child requires a stepped up language enrichment program coupled with appropriate support services from varied professional sources.

Therapy for Communication

The development of listening skills through auditory training is a significant part of a therapy program for children and adolescents with moderately severe to severe hearing losses. Speechreading is also a part of the total therapy plan that is intended to assist the hearing-impaired individual recognize facial expressions, gestures, and body movements, all of which contribute to the perception of speech. Although much has been done to investigate the value of speechreading, it is still a misunderstood concept. It is an error to believe that speechreading alone can replace hearing in the complete understanding of spoken discourse. It is also an error to believe that more than about 50 percent of the sounds of speech may be perceived through speechreading alone, therefore therapy with the hearing-impaired youngster must include auditory training along with speechreading for maximum benefit.

Besides assistance with hearing, auditory training, and speechreading, children who have hearing losses need help with the development of a communication system. Both oral and manual techniques are available, and the controversy between the use of oral-only versus manual-only communication methods is long-standing. This does not pose a problem for children who have moderately severe hearing losses because they can still speak intelligibly. The situation is different, however, for children with losses greater than 90 dB; they may have little understandable speech. Out of these two extremes has come a "total communication" philosophy that individualizes communication for each child using both manual and oral techniques when necessary. With this approach a child's language program may consist of a combination of amplification, natural gestures, pantomime, sign language, finger spelling, lip reading, and body language with or without oral speech. In other words, the child learns to use whatever tools provide the best possible means of communication.

Following the early intervention and management of young hearing-impaired children, the educational and social development of the youngster becomes of primary importance. The following chapter "Implications of Hearing Loss to Educational and Social Development . . ." is intended to provide information with regard to this challenge.

QUESTIONS FOR DISCUSSION

1. The human ear is made up of three parts; name them. What are their respective functions?
2. What kinds of information may be derived from the audiogram?
3. What kinds of problems may cause a conductive hearing loss? What may be done to alleviate such problems?
4. A severe hearing loss occurs between what dB levels? What are some causes of such a hearing loss?
5. Prelingual deafness refers to what kind of problem?
6. All infants and young children identified as at-risk for hearing loss should be followed up for further testing. Why is such early identification so important?
7. The basic audiologic test battery includes a variety of tests. What are their different functions?
8. Ventilating tubes are important because they may help alleviate conductive hearing losses. Why?
9. Auditory trainers may be utilized in the classroom. Why?
10. What is the teacher's role with respect to the hearing-impaired child?

REFERENCES

Berg F (1970). Definition and incidence. In F Berg & SG Fletcher (Eds.), *The hard of hearing child* (pp 7–12). Orlando, FL: Grune & Stratton

Eagles EL, Wishik SM, & Doerfler LG (1967). Hearing and sensitivity and ear disease in children: A prospective study [Monograph]. *Laryngoscope* 1–274

Jerger J (1980). Dissenting report: Mass impedance screening. *Annals of Otology, Rhinology, and Laryngology, 89* (Suppl. 69), 21–22

Klein JO (1978). Epidemiology of otitis media. In ER Harford, FH Bess, D Bluestone, & JO Klein (Eds.), *Impedance screening for middle ear disease in children* (pp 11–16). Orlando, FL: Grune & Stratton

Knauf VH (1978). Language and speech training. In J Katz (Ed.), *Handbook of clinical audiology* (pp 549–564). Baltimore: Williams & Wilkins

McFarland WH, Simmons FB, & Jones FR (1980). An automated hearing screening technique for newborns. *Journal of Speech and Hearing Disorders, 45,* 495–503

Northern JL, & Downs MP (1974). *Hearing in children.* Baltimore: Williams & Wilkins

Northern JL, & Downs MP (1978). *Hearing in children.* Baltimore: Williams & Wilkins

Northern JL, & Lemme M (1986). Hearing and auditory disorders. In GH Shames & EH Wiig (Eds.), *Human communication disorders* (pp 415–444). Columbus, OH: Charles E. Merrill

Ross M (1975). Hearing aids for young children. *Otolaryngology Clinics of North America, 8,* 125–141

Shulman-Galambos C, & Galambos R (1979). Brainstem evoked response audiometry in newborn hearing screening. *Archives of Otolaryngology, 105,* 86–90

Silverman SR, Lane HS, & Calvert DR (1978). Early and elementary education. In H Davis & SR Silverman (Eds.), *Hearing and Deafness* (4th ed.) (pp 384–425). New York: Holt, Rinehart, & Winston

Stewart JF (1979). Newborn infant hearing screening. A five-year pilot project. *Journal of Otolaryngology, 6,* 477–481

14

Implications of Hearing Loss to Educational and Social Development Including the Mainstreamed Educationally Deaf Child

Ralph G. Leverett
Allan O. Diefendorf

The Education for All Handicapped Children Act (Public Law 94-142) was signed into law in 1975. All children who are "handicapped" and in need of "special education" and "related services" must be identified, located, evaluated and assured a free, appropriate public education in the least restrictive environment. Appropriate management of children with auditory disorders lies within that directive.

The concept of least-restrictive environment and Public Law 94-142 has been interpreted differently by various state and local education agencies. As a result, a regular classroom teacher or a special educator certified in an area other than education of the deaf may become the major service provider for students with varying speech–language and hearing disorders and possibly, different communication systems.

This chapter seeks to provide suggestions for the instruction of hearing-impaired persons primarily within the public school context. The assumed audience includes the following preservice and inservice professionals: special educators with various certifications (especially those seeking certification in education of the deaf), regular educators who have become service providers for the hearing-impaired, and parents of the hearing-impaired.

ORAL COMMUNICATION PROBLEMS
IN CHILDREN AND ADOLESCENTS
Copyright © 1988 by Grune & Stratton, Inc.

MAINSTREAMING AND THE LEAST-RESTRICTIVE ENVIRONMENT

A definition of mainstreaming includes some concept of integration of exceptional students in the regular classroom. Common usage of the term probably includes anything from minimal integration to virtually complete integration of the student in regular education classes. We will assume that the term includes both ends of the continuum, but we lean toward the former use of that term—placement in the regular education classroom for any part of the school day.

It is quite possible for many hearing-impaired students to enter the mainstream in at least one subject area. Adequate cooperation between the regular and special education teacher makes this possible. Ideally, each should be committed to the task, and anything less than full commitment generally compromises the exceptional student's opportunities for learning.

Mainstreaming has failed often enough within the existing system that alternatives to a conventional mainstream have been offered. The conventional or traditional structure of the mainstream views students as possessing homogeneous skills. Students of the same chronologic age are seen as ready to learn the same objectives over the same time period across all curricular areas—hardly ideal for the exceptional learner.

A modification of the traditional structure would recognize students as the heterogeneous learners they are. As such they vary from one another in readiness to learn and in rate of learning, and they vary within themselves in their ability to progress in various curricular areas (Stainback, Stainback, Courtnage, & Jaben, 1985). Common pleas for similar restructuring of the schools have occurred with regularity over many years.

The concept of reverse mainstreaming also represents a departure from the norm. Although regular and special educators have practiced an "underground" system for many years, the practice has received recent professional support. McCann, Semmel, and Nevin (1985) reported 58 percent of regular educators in eight school districts sent one or more nonhandicapped students to special education classrooms for specific services (usually reading or math) or activities. This represents a mutually beneficial system that makes mainstreaming more acceptable to regular educators.

A more difficult educational dilemma is the choice of the least-restrictive environment. Public school service delivery options, ranked from least to most restrictive, include the regular classroom, itinerant services, resource rooms, and self-contained special-education classrooms. The authors urge a conservative interpretation of the least-restrictive environment. Financial pressures created by the need to educate all certifiable exceptional children have led school systems to economize in all possible areas. This has increased the number of students on the least-restrictive end of the service continuum. In other words, more students have been placed in regular classrooms, itinerant programs, or resource rooms away from the self-contained settings. Such practice seems to be in full compliance with the concept.

Placement of hearing-impaired students within the regular classroom assumes that adequate services will be available including the possible need for interpreters, notetakers, the services of an educational audiologist, and speech–language pathologists as the level of needs is determined. It also assumes a rather high level of independence on the part of the student. Essentially the same services and level of independence should be considered for students receiving itinerant services.

Students in resource rooms have the advantage of a very flexible system. Placement in this setting may result in arranged services approximating those of the itinerant teacher to those of the self-contained classroom. Teachers in this setting have the advantage of being stationed in one (sometimes two) schools, and the advantage of daily consults with regular classroom teachers. A certain emotional advantage allows the student to feel that educational and/or emotional support is easily obtained.

Self-contained classrooms may still be the least-restrictive environment for some hearing-impaired students. This is especially true for the students whose communication systems (aural/oral or manual) are being developed, or those who have a communication system that is inadequate for placement in one of the other service options.

Consultants are an additional option in some school systems; however, their role in service delivery is not universally accepted. Although this option seems ideally suited to public schools, especially whenever many students are placed in regular classrooms, the authors' experiences with this position suggest that the consultant frequently is resented as another professional who "tells me how to do my job" and who does not assume the responsibility of the classroom teacher.

The question of placement in the least-restrictive environment should be addressed as objectively as possible. The entire management team (M-team) should consider present needs. But future needs may be perceivable, and placement must consider as many of these as possible. The least-restrictive environment should be the place where the student can perform best and receives all necessary services, where academic tasks are within the range of abilities, and where communication and living skills can be developed to allow successful functioning within the post-school years.

Further, PL 94-142 made explicit the role of parents as full members of the educational teams. Teachers of the hearing-impaired need to inform parents of their legal rights as well as their children's educational rights.

TEACHERS AND THE HEARING-IMPAIRED

Teacher Competencies

Various state and professional organizations establish criteria for minimum certification of teachers of the hearing-impaired. Ninety-two competencies covering many aspects of preparation and abilities have been ranked by degree of importance (Mackie, 1956; Scott, 1983). Skills related to language development were ranked first in the Mackie 1956 study; whereas first in the Scott 1983 study was the ability to recognize and provide for the differences of each pupil. Each of these reflects the historical aspects of their respective studies. Other emphases ranked among the top five in both studies were the ability to meet the social needs of students (in adapting to school and society) and the importance of establishing socially acceptable standards of personal hygiene and behavior. Generally, the more recent study indicated a shift from a speech instruction emphasis toward working as a team member to meet the individual needs of the student.

Schow and Nerbonne (1980) mention additional teacher competencies. These include skills necessary to read hearing aid specification sheets, the ability to serve in a variety of possible roles in speech habilitation, training sufficient to teach both hearing-impaired and deaf students, and "the major responsibilities of educators of the hearing impaired"—to ensure the proper function of hearing aids and related equipment.

EDUCATIONAL SPECIALISTS AND THE HEARING-IMPAIRED

The Educational Audiologist

The role of the educational audiologist may include initial identification of students referred to the program, ongoing assessment of students within the program, maintenance of hearing aids and classroom amplification systems, and cooperative habilitation/rehabilitation efforts (with the special educator). Consultation with parents and regular educators, and the presentation of workshops to a variety of professionals within and outside the school system may also be included as responsibilities.

The Aural Rehabilitator

Closely related to the role of the educational audiologist is that of the aural rehabilitator. Similar responsibilities exist in the roles of these two professionals and that of the teacher of the hearing-impaired.

The variation of roles probably represents a concentration on different aspects of the educational process. Schow and Nerbonne (1980) list concerns with teaming, seating, visual aids, reduction of classroom noise, and choosing language training systems among the responsibilities of the aural rehabilitator in addition to providing actual hearing and speech therapy. Again, these certainly are concerns of the other two professionals, and the roles are destined to overlap at times.

Interpreters in the Classroom

Interpreters should possess good memory, adequate facial and body language, facility in spoken and signed messages of the hearing-impaired, the ability to orally interpret and translate, mastery of sign vocabulary and language structure, and the ability to simultaneously interpret and translate.

Additional requirements would include the social skills of diplomacy and cooperation. These persons must work in tandem with classroom teachers. They may need to request outlines of material, reference books, and clarification of teachers' objectives. The ability to be useful to the hearing-impaired student and unobtrusive to the remainder of the class is also desirable.

Notetakers should possess many of the characteristics of the interpreter. Basic qualifications include above average academic ability, sensitivity to the needs of the hearing-impaired, ability to accept direction and/or criticism, and knowledge of subject matter. This last qualification implies that the notetaker not be a student within the classroom. However, strong students usually make above average notetakers. They have the additional advantage of serving as practical tutors for homework and exams.

Wilson (1982) suggests three sources of notetakers: volunteers, paraprofessionals, and professionals. Each has advantages and disadvantages. The no-cost advantage of volunteers is countered by the need to provide training and monitoring of performance. Professionals possess training and require virtually no monitoring for accuracy, but the cost may be greater than the cost of paraprofessionals who require occasional accuracy and performance evaluations.

CLASSROOM CONSIDERATIONS

Instructional Views

Assessment

The last decade has witnessed a move away from test bias and toward fairness in the evaluation of hearing-impaired children. These changes were mandated by federal law, but also reflect the desires of school personnel to apply assessment results more directly to classroom instruction. Many norm-referenced tests have been redesigned or restandardized, and the use of criterion-referenced instruments has increased in response to the need to be both "honest" and "relevant" in evaluation.

What factors should be considered in the evaluation of hearing-impaired persons? Ziezula (1982) listed four major concerns: the nature of the test items (verbal or performance), the language requirements to understand directions, discriminatory items related to auditory dysfunction, and whether hearing-impaired persons were included in the standardization of a test.

Beyond these general questions are those related to the administration of the test or test battery. The diagnostician should be aware of various blocks to communication. From the diagnostician's standpoint, speech intelligibility and the need to simplify test language are of primary importance for the aural-oral student. Related to this would be checks of auditory equipment (proper functioning of hearing aids or auditory trainers) and a remembrance of the limitations of speechreading (Hargrove & Poteet, 1984). Awareness of language limitations (both vocabulary and concepts), notation of any departures from standardized test procedure, a natural speaking pattern, and the knowledge that test scores will generally be lower than the student's true ability are also among the skills the examiner should apply to an evaluation.

Individualizing Instruction (II)

Contrary to its apparent meaning, II does not require one-to-one instruction, one teacher, one child. Stevens and Rosenshine (1981) consider it appropriate to several formats; small groups, regular classroom presentations, and occasional one-to-one instruction. Critical to individualization is material that results in a high percentage of accuracy. A well-placed, well-paced student in any classroom with materials appropriate to his or her academic levels meets the requirements of individualization.

Students who do poorly in mainstream settings may be placed beyond their ability levels. Again, the least-restrictive environment should be considered carefully. Neither the teacher nor the student should be burdened with the task. Students placed in the least-restrictive environment allow teachers to continue teaching with only minor modification in presentation or material.

Adapting Instruction

Instruction can be generally modified along three lines: adjustments in materials, in instruction, and in requirements (Lewis & Doorlag, 1983). This often means that the teacher may go a step or two beyond the normal preparation for and implementation of instruction.

Modification of materials often includes the altering of sequence (chapters may be rearranged), simplifying the written directions of workbooks, the addition of prompts (underlining, highlighting, circling, etc.), and error analysis of homework and tests.

Teaching procedures can be altered by making assignments and instructions very explicit, and by altering the pace of instruction. Guided and independent practice provides the student additional time to master activities and the remediation of skills not fully developed. Guided practice is carefully monitored work in which the teacher works on an almost individual level for the introduction of material. Once the student seems comfortable with the task, independent practice is introduced. In this stage the student's work is still carefully monitored but less often and with less direct contact with the teacher. Each of these stages moves the student toward independent work, and remediation or reinstruction may occur at any stage.

Task requirements may be tailored to the student's needs in a least three ways: changing the criteria for successful performance, allowing the use of various visual aids, or by breaking the task into smaller units. Changing the criteria for success may involve granting a longer time for mastery or changing the percentage of correct answers required for mastery. Visual aids such as wall charts, timelines taped to the student's desk, the use of "counters" or calculators, and any of several other supports have value for "weak" students. These modifications should always be considered less than ideal adjustments. They are artificial aids to learning, but experience indicates they are necessary for some students who may never function on a truly independent level. These modifications as well as others have been discussed in greater detail by Lewis and Doorlag (1983).

Mastery Learning

Mastery learning (Bloom, 1971; Carroll, 1971) presents a method of instruction that is based on small units of materials and clear objectives and teaching strategies. Brief diagnostic tests are prepared for each unit, and supplementary instruction is built into the program. In this manner, remediation of unmastered material is carried out until mastery is achieved. Virtually any subject area can be adapted to mastery learning principles.

Mastery of the task is seen in relationship to time, student effort, quality of instruction, the student's ability to comprehend, and his or her aptitude. Seen in this light, educators and students share accountability for learning.

Instrumental Enrichment

Instrumental enrichment (Feuerstein, 1980) assumes that "mediated learning" occurs whenever a culture bearer (parent, teacher, friend) more or less interprets the world to a younger person. Not only are events pointed out to the younger person, but the meaning of these events is also discussed. If we simplify the "persons and events" to a school setting, we have a teacher–learner relationship that, if adequate, results in a genuine learning experience. If in some manner this relationship is faulty, we have a breakdown in transmitting the "culture of school" with all of its information to the learner.

Our purpose in devoting a section to instrumental enrichment is to stimulate interest in the program. Its carefully constructed units, its attempts to "bridge" between the knowledge the learner brings to a new learning encounter and its deliberate approach to teaching generalization to academics and the broader world, are worth investigation. Keane (1985), Rohr-Redding (1985), and Martin (1984) suggest successful application of this program to education for the hearing-impaired. They report improvement in student performance and revitalized teachers.

Learning-Disabled Hearing-Impaired Students

Caution should always be exercised before any labeling of children. However, teachers have long recognized that some hearing-impaired students appear to have learning characteristics different from those apparently related to "just" diminished hearing. La Sasso (1985) warned against the overinterpretation of characteristics similar to learning disabilities. She suggested that lack of progress in some hearing-impaired students may be attributable to poorly developed curricula, inadequate instruction, and faulty pacing of students through the curricula. Further, she indicated that "for most deaf children," learning problems are due to the limitations of language, inadequate communication skills, poor inferencing abilities, and a lack of general word knowledge. She suggested the use of more "specific, less ambiguous terms" such as "visual perceptual problem" or "visual memory problem" to describe the learning limitations of these students. Such terms, however, are also commonly used to identify specific deficits in certified learning-disabled students.

Whether learning-disabled hearing-impaired students exist or not may always be debatable. Research at the University of Kansas has suggested that hearing "low achievers" and learning-disabled students at the secondary level share several learning problems (Deshler, Schumaker, Alley, Warner, & Clark, 1982). This study provides a framework for considering the possibility of a learning-disabled hearing-impaired population, especially within secondary-school settings.

The shift from elementary classrooms to secondary classrooms involves several dramatic changes in the environment, and therefore affects the student in that environment. Secondary teachers assume a greater level of independence among students. Instruction is heavily weighted toward the lecture method, and few aids are provided to help students organize information received orally or assigned as homework. The language structure of the classroom becomes more complex, and few comprehension checks are made. Students are less likely to be asked to demonstrate knowledge verbally while written communication skills are taxed more heavily. Additionally, the assumed ability to work independently results in more seatwork (47 percent of the time). Class discussion and audiovisual aids in the Deshler et al. study were each used only 10 percent of the time.

These findings fit easily into either side of the issue of learning-disabled hearing-impaired students. Surely they emphasize with equal importance the concerns of La Sasso (1985). They also suggest that "low achievers," regardless of the reasons for low achievement, will almost certainly have difficulty in the secondary setting without substantial academic support. Perhaps the significance of this research, then, is not whether a subset of hearing-impaired students exists, but rather that we should carefully consider the placement of "weak" hearing-impaired students in regular classrooms or in an itinerant program as the least-restrictive environment at any educational level. Self-contained programs for the hearing-impaired at the secondary level may be rarer than those at the elementary level, but we are responsible for providing appropriate education at either level.

Reading and Related Matters

Trybus and Karchmer (1977) found reading comprehension scores of 9-year-old deaf students to be at second-grade level. Scores of 20 year olds were only three years above the second-grade level. In a related study, Jenesma (1975) analyzed achievement test scores of 6,873 children with hearing losses significant enough to require special education. Within this group of students ages 6–19, 14 year olds functioned at a third-grade level in reading. Certainly factors such as age of onset and the degree of training following identification of a hearing loss are significant in determining achievement in language-related areas. However, reading and related language arts activities generally pose significant problems for the hearing-impaired student in almost any type of special education setting.

Suggestions for Classroom Management

A review of a dozen or more survey texts in Special Educati_
able similarity in recommendations for classroom management of the ɪɪᴄ
impaired. Blankenship and Lilly (1981) have, perhaps, the most complete summary
of recommendations. Those discussed in this chapter generally represent the most
well established.

Preferential Seating

Preferential seating is perhaps the most obvious thing to do. It includes not only
seating the student near the teacher and chalkboard, but also seating the student so
the better ear is directed away from interfering noise sources. Consider such critical
factors as the acoustics of the classroom (signal-to-noise ratio) and reverberation
(amount of echo in the room).

Face-to-Face Contact

The teacher should not feel so restricted as to move artificially or awkwardly
about the room. Awareness of the need for visual cues in speech reading, however,
suggests that this is important. One method of reducing the awkwardness is to use
an overhead projector. This provides the benefits of a chalkboard and the necessary
facial view.

Natural Speaking Manner

Natural speaking manner means just what it says. Use normal tones, gestures,
and lip movements. An exaggerated manner tires the teacher and will not be
beneficial to the student.

Avoid Backlighting

Generally backlighting means standing in front of windows or any other light
source. The glare makes it difficult for students to see speech movements and facial
expressions.

Provide Graphic Cues

A reminder to illustrate concepts, new vocabulary, directions, and other orally
presented material is hardly necessary. But, the teacher is encouraged to go beyond
the normal degree of graphic supplements to the oral presentation.

Materials and Instructions Appropriate to the Child's Level

Teachers of all students quickly realize the need to modify commercial materials and to supplement "basic materials" with a variety of similar materials written on
several levels. Generally, hearing-impaired students will function several grades
below that expected for grade placement or chronologic age.

Comprehension Checks

Comprehension checks are especially important for information presented
orally. Hearing-impaired children frequently "fake" comprehension. A reasonably

accurate check of comprehension can be made by having students repeat the information you have presented rather than simply asking if they understand. Problems in this area are generally related to language comprehension, not intelligence.

Buddy System

Whenever more formal notetakers are unavailable, a student in good academic standing may be chosen to take additional notes (carbon-tissue sets makes this no additional effort). The buddy also serves to help the student to locate in-class assignments and to follow oral instruction. Most classes will include several volunteers. Both the volunteers and student being served should have the freedom to alter the arrangement if the "pairing" ceases to be productive.

Concern for Idiomatic Language

Teachers should be aware that hearing-impaired students often literalize idioms. Awareness of this allows the teacher to interpret figurative language. Written materials should be reviewed for use of any potentially misunderstood concepts. Additionally, teachers may need to clarify their spoken idiomatic expressions.

Awareness of the Limitations of Amplification

Included here is awareness of the true characteristics of hearing aids—that *all* sound is amplified and may compete with the speech signal. Basic trouble-shooting skills will allow teachers to be alert for dead batteries and broken cords or tone hooks and receivers. Spare cords/tone hooks and batteries are a must for the classroom.

Bells, Signals, and Alarms

Students may need to learn the precise meaning of these frequent interruptions and, additionally, the responses to them. A student serving as a buddy can be helpful in this area of adjustment, but teachers should continue to alert students to the unexpected.

Music Classes

With some adjustment in requirements many hearing-impaired students can profit from music classes, a part of the regular curriculum. Attempts should be made to include them in these activities. It is important to remember that although the understanding of speech may be poor, students may have skills useful in recognizing and appreciating rhythm patterns.

Preassignments

Formal classroom interpreters and virtually all concerned parents will profit from "knowing what comes next." This is especially true in courses with significant reading assignments. Being able to work ahead allows the hearing-impaired student to keep pace with the hearing peers. Preintroduction to new concepts and vocabulary will be particularly helpful.

Modified Testing Format

Creative teachers will learn modifications that do not compromise their expectations. Among the more common modifications are increasing the length of time allowed for tests and allowing interpreters to translate printed concepts to sign equivalents. The language of directions may be as difficult for the hearing-impaired student as the question itself. Directions and questions may need to be written in simpler language and examples given to guide the student.

Captioned Films

All teachers may profit from the use of captioned films. The captions may actually provide information useful to hearing persons with faulty listening skills. A large variety of captioned films and videotapes is available including commercial movies and vocationally oriented material.

A Final Word About Classrooms

The effective use of bulletin boards can be an excellent supplement to instruction. They are especially useful in providing a visual documentation of the components of the unit. The teacher may begin with a board on which only the title of the unit has been placed. As the elements of the unit are introduced, visual representations (pictures, symbols, and completed seat work assignments) may be added. This provides information useful in the introduction and discussion of the subject matter, and by the unit's completion, an automatic review of that material fills the bulletin board.

Finally, open discussion of the effects of hearing loss may prepare hearing peers for the hearing-impaired student and increase the chance of the hearing-impaired student's school acceptance. Additional discussion of the limitations of a hearing aid should be included. Provisions can be made for hearing students to listen to a hearing aid to create some empathy (not sympathy) for the user. Typically, hearing students are eager to learn about the implications of hearing loss and may request classes in sign language to better communicate with students who use that system.

The classroom considerations and suggestions for management are intended to make the regular educator more comfortable with hearing-impaired students in their classroom. Most important, however, is the teacher's willingness and openness to work with the exceptional learner and various support personnel.

QUESTIONS FOR DISCUSSION

1. Discuss Public Law 94-142 and its impact on education.
2. Explain "least-restrictive environment," and discuss examples of what environment is appropriate for children and adolescents with varying degrees of educational difficulties.
3. Discuss the roles of different educational specialists in the classroom.

4. Discuss the controversy surrounding "learning-disabled hearing-impaired students."
5. List and discuss competencies that teachers of the hearing-impaired should possess.
6. Explain why the concept of preferential seating is important to the hearing-impaired student.
7. What factors lead to poor reading skills in hearing-impaired and deaf students?
8. Discuss how "adapting instruction" could be utilized in the classroom for hearing-impaired students.
9. List and discuss the components of mastery learning.
10. Discuss the major limitations of a personal hearing aid in a noisy environment.

REFERENCES

Blankenship C, & Lilly M (1981). *Mainstreaming students with learning and behavior problems: Techniques for the classroom teacher.* New York: Holt, Rinehart, and Winston

Bloom B (1971). Mastery learning. In J Block (Ed.), *Mastery learning: Theory and practice* (pp 47–63). New York: Holt, Rinehart, and Winston

Carroll J (1971). Problems of measurement related to the concept of learning for mastery. In J Block (Ed.), *Mastery learning: Theory and practice* (pp 29–46). New York: Holt, Rinehart, and Winston

Deshler D, Schumaker J, Alley G, Warner M, & Clark F (1982). Learning disabilities in adolescent and young adult populations: Research implications. *Focus on Exceptional Children, 15* (1), 1–12

Feuerstein R (1980). *Instrumental enrichment: An intervention program for cognition modificability.* Baltimore: University Park Press

Hargrove L, & Poteet J (1984). *Assessment in special education: The education evaluation.* Englewood Cliffs, NJ: Prentice-Hall

Jenesma C (1975). *The relationship between academic achievement and the demographic characteristics of hearing impaired children and youth.* Washington, D.C.: Gallaudet College, Office of Demographic Studies

Keane K (1985). Application of Feuerstein's mediated learning construct to deaf persons. In D Martin (Ed.), *Cognition, education, and deafness: Directions for research and instruction* (pp 141–145). Washington, D.C.: Gallaudet College Press

La Sasso C (1985). Learning disabilities: Let's be careful before labeling deaf children. *Perspectives for Teachers of the Hearing Impaired, 3* (5), 2–4

Lewis R, & Doorlag D (1983). *Teaching special students in the mainstream.* Columbus, OH: Charles E. Merrill

Mackie R (1956). *Teachers of children who are deaf* (Bulletin No. 6). Washington, D.C.: U.S. Department of Health, Education, and Welfare

Martin D (1984). Cognitive modification for the hearing impaired adolescent: The promise. *Exceptional Children, 51* (3), 235–242

McCann S, Semmel M, & Nevin A (1985). Reverse mainstreaming: Nonhandicapped students in special education classrooms. *RASE, 6* (1), 13–19

Rohr-Redding C (1985). Can thinking skills be incorporated into a curriculum? In D Martin

(Ed.), *Cognition, education, and deafness: Directions for research and instruction* (pp 168–171). Washington, D.C.: Gallaudet College Press

Schow R, & Nerbonne M (1980). *Introduction to aural rehabilitation.* Austin: Pro-Ed

Scott P (1983). Have competencies needed by teachers of the hearing impaired changed in 25 years? *Exceptional Children, 50* (1), 48–53

Stainback W, Stainback S, Courtnage L, & Jaben T (1985). Facilitating mainstreaming by modifying the mainstream. *Exceptional Children, 52* (2), 144–152

Stevens R, & Rosenshine B (1981). Advances in research on teaching. *Exceptional Education Quarterly, 2* (1), 1–9

Trybus R, & Karchmer G (1977). School achievement scores of hearing impaired children: National data on achievement status and growth patterns. *American Annals of the Deaf, 122,* 35–53

Wilson J (1982). Tutoring and notetaking as classroom support services for the deaf student. In D Sims, G Walter & R Whitehead (Eds.), *Deafness and communication: Assessment and training,* (pp 407–415). Baltimore: Williams and Wilkins

Ziezula F (Ed.). (1982). *Assessment of hearing-impaired people: A guide for selecting psychological, educational, and vocational tests.* Washington, D.C.: Gallaudet College Press

INDEX

Page numbers in *italics* indicate illustrations. Page numbers followed by *t* indicate tables.

A

Academic language, 49
Acoustic immittance in screening school-age children, for hearing impairment, 140
Additions
  definition of, 122
  as misarticulations, 116–117
Adenoidectomy, hypernasality after, 11
Adenoids, enlarged, problems from, 10–11
Age
  articulation development and, 112*t*, 113
  language and listening as function of, 45
Air conduction tests in hearing assessment, 141–142
Alarms, adjustment to, for hearing-impaired, 160
American Speech-Language-Hearing Association (ASHA), certification by, 18
Amplification for hearing impairment, 145–147
  awareness of limitations of, 160
Ann Arbor decision, 68–70
Articulation, 111–122
  definition of, 122
  development of
    factors related to, 113–114
    normal, 112*t*, 113
    normal versus abnormal, 5
  speech, improvement program and, 114–115

therapy for, stuttering control through, 103
Articulation disorders, 3, 7, 115–118
  additions as, 116–117
  causes of, 117–118
  in cerebral palsy, 117
  distortions as, 116
  in emotionally disturbed, 118
  functional, 117
  introduction to, 36–37
  linguistic disorders and, 118
  in mentally retarded, 117–118
  omissions as, 116
  organic, 117
  prevention of, 113–115
  substitutions as, 115–116
  treatment of, 118–120
    classroom teacher in, 120–122
    distinctive feature theory of, 119
    early theories and their applications in, 119
    motokinesthetic method of, 119
    phonologic approach to, 120
    recent theories and their applications in, 120
    wedge approach to, 120
  types of, 115
Articulators
  definition of, 123
  structure of, articulation development and, 113–114
Assessment, language-impaired student identification by, 46–48
Ataxia in cerebral palsy, 10
Athetosis in cerebral palsy, 10

165